AN INTRODUC
FOR THE

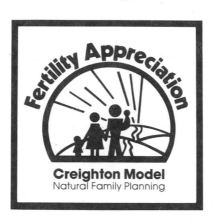

Creighton Model
Natural Family Planning

THE OVULATION METHOD
OF NATURAL FAMILY PLANNING

Thomas W. Hilgers, M.D.
Dip. ABOG, ABLS, SRS

With an Introduction to NaProTechnology
The Contemporary Approach to Women's Health Care

POPE PAUL VI INSTITUTE PRESS
OMAHA, NE 68106

International Standard Book Number: 0-9626485-2-3
Libary of Congress Catalogue Card Number: 92-81747

Cover design by Susan Parrish

THIRD EDITION

Published by **POPE PAUL VI INSTITUTE PRESS**
6901 MERCY ROAD
OMAHA, NEBRASKA 68106 USA

ABOUT THE AUTHOR

Thomas W. Hilgers, M.D., Dip. ABOG, ABLS, SRS, is the director of the Pope Paul VI Institute for the Study of Human Reproduction in Omaha, Nebraska. He began his first research in natural family planning in 1968 as a senior medical student. Working at St. Louis University Natural Family Planning Center, St. Louis, Missouri and the Creighton University Natural Family Planning Education and Research Center, Omaha, Nebraska, he and his co-workers, developed the Creighton Model Natural Family Planning System. Those intrinsically involved in the development of this system, along with Dr. Hilgers, were Ann M. Prebil, RN, BSN, CNFPE; K. Diane Daly, RN, CNFPE and Susan K. Hilgers, BS, CNFPE.

Currently, Dr. Hilgers is a Senior Medical Consultant in Obstetrics, Gynecology and Reproductive Medicine at the Pope Paul VI Institute for the Study of Human Reproduction and the director of the Institute's National Center for the Treatment of Reproductive Disorders.

TABLE OF CONTENTS

INTRODUCTION

Our work began in 1976 as an independent evaluation of the Ovulation Method of Natural Family Planning which had first been described by the Drs. John and Lyn Billings in Melbourne, Australia. As we progressed in our work, we were able to independently verify that the claims made by the Drs. Billings were correct and that this method of family planning had many outstanding features to it.

As we undertook our scientific investigations, we were able to solidify the scientific foundations of the method. In addition, we were able to develop a teaching methodology which has now become known as the Creighton Model Natural Family Planning System.

This is a standardized teaching system which is used throughout the United States and in several foreign countries. Because it is standardized, there is a common language that all couples use making the entire system very objective.

Creighton Model Natural Family Planning services are provided by Natural Family Planning Practitioners (NFPP) who are trained in a 13 month allied health course. Eventually, they become certified through the American Academy of Natural Family Planning, the national certifying body.

Not only is this method an excellent one for reliably achieving and avoiding pregnancy, it is also an excellent system for assisting couples in the expansion of their human sexuality horizons. By understanding our fertility and by periodically avoiding genital contact (if it is the desire to avoid pregnancy), one is challenged to explore the other, non-genital ways of sexually interacting. This has the effect of broadening the basis of the relationship and the commitments of that relationship. Indeed, it is a system which requires mutual love, cooperation and commitment and these are the ingredients that lead to a *bonded marriage*.

Thus, the teachers are very well trained to assist you in all aspects of method use including problem solving and case management.

The most recent research with this method has shown it to be not only an excellent method of family planning, but also an incredible method for *gynecologic and reproductive health maintenance.*

This method, being based on the presence or absence of the cervical mucus discharge, is based on the presence of very sensitive *biomarkers*. These include the menstrual flow and other bleeding episodes, dry days and days in which mucus is present. When one understands these patterns—through good record keeping— and one is in contact with a well-trained Natural Family Planning Practitioner, one can monitor one's reproductive health in a way that has simply never been available before.

Using the Creighton Model as a means of monitoring reproductive health has lead to a new reproductive science called NaProTechnology. This science uses the patterns of mucus discharge and bleeding in such a way that it allows for the interpretation of various health events. Instead of suppressing or destroying fertility, as is so common in today's world, it *cooperates* with the normal reproductive systems. Thus, NaProTechnology refers to a good understanding of the *natural procreative systems.*

In this third edition, I have added a chapter entitled "An Introduction to NaProTechnology." This chapter gives a review on how this method can be used in a variety of different reproductive health related areas.

This natural family planning system *is really incredible.* While maintaining your integrity and preserving your choices with regard to the use of the natural phases of fertility and infertility, you also have the extraordinary benefit of being able to monitor your gynecologic and reproductive health throughout your life. It is a system which really *empowers women* to take charge of their reproductive health and be an equal partner in evaluating it and maintaining it.

We hope that your experience with the Creighton Model Natural Family Planning System is an outstanding one.

Thomas W. Hilgers, M.D., Dip. ABOG, ABLS, SRS
Senior Medical Consultant
Obstetrics, Gynecology & Reproductive Medicine
Director, Pope Paul VI Institute
    for the Study of Human Reproduction

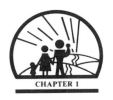
THE OVULATION METHOD

The *Ovulation Method of Natural Family Planning* was first described by Drs. John and Lyn Billings in Melbourne, Australia. It is a *unique* method of natural family planning. This method relies upon a sign - the *discharge of cervical mucus* - which is *essential to human fertility*. Because of this, the Ovulation Method is the *most precise* of all natural methods.

The purpose of this booklet is to *introduce you* to the Ovulation Method. It *does not* replace adequate instruction in the method. The booklet is specifically designed for use in association with an adequate instructional experience provided by a properly trained natural family planning practitioner (NFPP) or natural family planning instructor (NFPI) who has a thorough grasp of the principles outlined in this booklet and its associated teaching materials.

NATURAL FAMILY PLANNING

The American Academy of Natural Family Planning defines natural family planning as a couple's understanding, acceptance and use of their phases of fertility and infertility for the purposes of achieving or avoiding pregnancy. Natural family planning is a way of embracing responsibility for love and life while maintaining the integrity of the couple's unitive and procreative abilities.

FERTILITY APPRECIATION

Fertility appreciation is the foundation of natural family planning. It is the ability of a couple to mutually *value, respect* and *understand* their fertility. Many couples find that the love and respect each holds for the other grows as their understanding and appreciation of their fertility grows. It accepts fertility as a normal and healthy process which is a precious gift from God; a gift to be loved, respected, understood and wisely used.

THE OVULATION METHOD

The circle diagram shown in Figure 1-1 illustrates the use of the Ovulation Method. The menstrual cycle begins with the first day of menstruation and ends with the day before the beginning of the next menstruation. The menstrual flow usually lasts from three to seven days. The first few days of menstruation are usually heavier in flow than the last few days.

After the cessation of the menstrual flow, the woman usually observes the absence of discharge or the presence of a dry sensation at the opening of the vagina.

After the dry days, there begins a discharge of cervical mucus which is usually *sticky, cloudy* or *tacky, cloudy*. After a few days, the mucus discharge progresses to become *clear, stretchy or lubricative. The last day of* mucus discharge that is clear, stretchy or lubricative is called *the Peak day.*

1

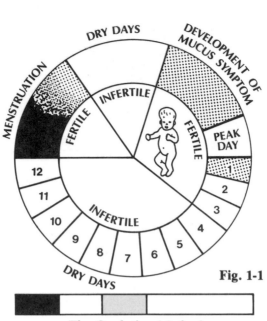

Fig. 1-1

The Ovulation Method

Following *the Peak day,* there is a *dramatic change* in the nature of the discharge. The discharge becomes sticky, cloudy or tacky, cloudy again or dry. The identification of the Peak day usually takes place one or two days following its actual occurrence. From the fourth day after the Peak until the beginning of the next menstrual flow, the woman is usually dry again.

All of the observations of the mucus are made at the opening of the vagina. Internal examinations should not be done.

The days of fertility in the Ovulation Method include the days of the menstrual flow and from the beginning of the mucus discharge through three days after the Peak day. The days of infertility in the method include the dry days following menstruation and from the fourth day after the Peak until the beginning of the next menstruation (See Chapters 6 for *basic method instructions* and the Appendix for *special circumstances).*

In the circle diagram you will notice that the days from the Peak day until the beginning of the next menstruation are numbered from 1 through 12. On the other hand, no such numbers appear for that phase of the cycle from the beginning of menstruation until the Peak. It is the preovulatory phase of the cycle which is highly variable in its length and the postovulatory phase of the cycle which is stable in its length. The *Peak day* has been shown to correlate very closely with the time of ovulation. Therefore, the time from the observation of the *Peak* until the beginning of the next menstruation is quite predictable. Knowing this will help you develop confidence in your observation of the Peak day and your use of the Ovulation Method.

The menstrual period is considered fertile because *every* woman will, on occasion, have a *short menstrual cycle.* When this occurs, *ovulation will occur earlier* than usual within the cycle. In such situations, there will be no dry days following menstruation. Mucus will be present during the menstrual flow and the conditions for sperm survival are right for a pregnancy to occur. Since no one can predict in advance when the menstrual

2

cycle will be short and since the Ovulation Method is a prospective method which does not rely upon past cycle history, the menstrual period is considered fertile.

The count of three days following the *Peak day* is necessary because ovulation can occur during these days. On average, ovulation occurs on the day of the *Peak*. However, ovulation may occur on the first, second or third day after the Peak.

ADVANTAGES OF THE OVULATION METHOD

There are many advantages to the Ovulation Method and they can be listed as follows:
- It is medically safe
- It is highly reliable
- It is morally acceptable
- It is easy to learn
- It is inexpensive
- It is highly versatile - it can be used at any stage of a woman's reproductive life
- It precisely identifies the true days of fertility and infertility
- It is a valuable aid for couples who are having difficulty in achieving pregnancy

THE IDEAL METHOD OF FAMILY PLANNING

In addition to the above advantages, the following make this an ideal method of family planning:

Shared Responsibility

Unlike contraceptives, the use of this method is equally shared by both the man and the woman. Couples learn to understand their combined fertility.

A True Method of Family Planning

The same method can be used to both achieve and avoid pregnancy making it a true method of family plannning.

Enhances One's Sexuality

The couple learns that true sexuality is spiritual, physical, intellectual, creative *and* emotional (S-P-I-C-E) in its dimensions. The use of natural family planning assists the couple in developing a balance to their sexual lives.

Loving Cooperation

The method helps build more loving cooperation in the important matters of sexuality and family planning. Couple's who practice natural family planning testify to the importance of periodically avoiding genital contact in the growth of their marriage relationship.

YOUR NATURAL FAMILY PLANNING TEACHER

Natural Family Planning services are delivered by educating the couple about their fertility. This is accomplished through a network of service programs developed and operated by specialists in natural family planning education. These specialists have received their education through a program whose professional curriculum was developed at the Creighton University Natural Family Planning Education and Research Center,

Creighton University School of Medicine, Omaha, Nebraska. Additional details about this training can be obtained directly from your teacher.

THE LEARNING SCHEDULE

The learning schedule is designed to meet the individual needs of each new client couple who enter the natural family planning program. Adequate instruction is *essential* for gaining confidence in the method and obtaining the maximum effectiveness possible. The couple *enters* the program with an *introductory session* and continues in the program with a series of individualized *follow-up* teaching appointments.

The introductory session: The introductory session is a slide presentation which *introduces* interested couples to the use of the Ovulation Method. It is a general presentation usually given to a small group of couples. An individual introductory session can be scheduled if the need arises. One can register for the introductory session by contacting the natural family planning center in your area.

Individualized follow-up sessions: Follow-up sessions are designed to *teach* couples to be actual users of the method. Personal instruction on the use of the method, as well as complete chart review, are services provided at the individual follow-up sessions which are scheduled at regular intervals. These individual follow-up sessions are *couple oriented* thus, both husband and wife should plan to participate in them. After the introduction session, the follow-up sessions occur in the following basic schedule:

    1st Follow-up------two weeks
    2nd Follow-up------four weeks
    3rd Follow-up------six weeks
    4th Follow-up------eight weeks
    5th Follow-up------three months
    6th Follow-up------six months
    7th Follow-up------nine months
    8th Follow-up------twelve months

Subsequent follow-ups are recommended every six to twelve months as you need them. The professional natural family planning teacher is also available for your consultation between sessions should any questions arise.

SUCCESSFUL USE OF THE METHOD

In order to use the method successfully, it is necessary to *make accurate observations* and to *chart them correctly. In addition, it is necessary to follow the instructions* of the method which depend upon the couple's decision to either achieve or avoid pregnancy. It is fundamental to the proper use of the method to realize that it is a *shared method of family planning.* The responsibility for its use is equally upon both the husband and the wife. For this, it is necessary to be mutually motivated in its use and to enter into its use with a loving and cooperative spirit.

Information contained in this booklet will be *useful to any couple* who wishes to use this method. As you begin to put your *time, energy and patience* into learning this method, keep in mind that it is an *investment in your future.*

CHAPTER 2

BASIC ANATOMY AND PHYSIOLOGY

It is important for all couples who use the Ovulation Method to have a basic understanding of how their bodies work. It is the purpose of this chapter to describe the basic anatomy and physiology of the human reproductive system. If the couple understands these few basic concepts, they will see how it applies later as they learn and use the Ovulation Method.

Let us begin by stating that *men are always fertile*. A man's fertility begins at the age of twelve or thirteen years and continues for the remainder of his life. It is a very important realization for men to appreciate the nature of their fertility. Men must understand their role in the fertility process if the Ovulation Method is to be successful.

The cell of human reproduction which is contributed by the male is called the *sperm*. Figure 2-1 shows an actual microscopic photograph of a sperm. The genetic material for reproduction is contained in the head of the sperm and the ability of the sperm to move from one place to the next comes from the motion of its tail.

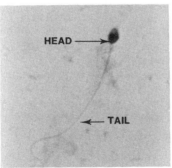

Fig. 2-1 This is an actual microscopic photograph of the sperm with its head and tail labelled.

The sperm are produced in two glands called the *testes* or *testicles* (Figure 2-2). The testicles are located on the outside of the male's body. They are located there primarily because the sperm are highly sensitive to heat and if the testes were located inside the body the increased temperature would destroy the sperm. On occasion, that may be a cause of male infertility. After the sperm are produced in the testicles they are transported along a tube called the *vas deferens*. From the vas deferens, the sperm go to the urethra and are transported to the outside of the male's body. The urethra is the channel which normally connects the bladder to the outside of the body.

While men are always fertile, women are, for the most part, infertile. Women are fertile for only a short period of time during each menstrual cycle. Of course, it is not entirely proper to talk about the man's fertility and the woman's fertility separately. The only meaningful point of discus-

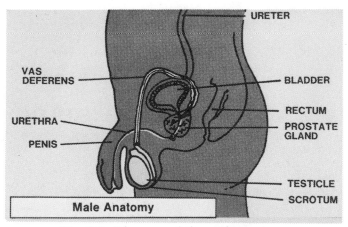

Fig. 2-2 Diagram of the male anatomy

sion is the *combined fertility* of the couple. Since women are for the most part infertile, this means that the couple for the most part is also infertile. Since men are always "fertile" and women are for the most part "infertile", the understanding of the couple's fertility is focused by necessity upon the cyclic variations of fertility and infertility that occur in the woman.

The reproductive organs of the woman lie within the protection of the pelvic cavity. In Figure 2-3, the location of the reproductive organs - the uterus, tubes and ovaries - are shown as they exist in the pelvis. Unlike the male, the reproductive organs in the woman are located inside the body.

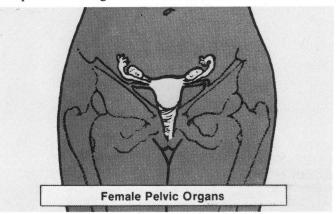

Fig. 2-3 The female pelvic organs

This cyclic variation of a woman's fertility is one of the most marvelously sophisticated events in all of nature. Indeed, it is a finely tuned, well-balanced system. The events are outwardly visible by the regular occurrence of menstruation and the characteristic flow of cervical mucus.

Figure 2-4 shows a diagram of the uterus, tubes and ovaries. The *ovaries* are almond shaped organs located on each side of the uterus. The *uterus* is basically a muscle which is pear shaped. There is a cavity within the uterus and at its opening there is an organ called the *cervix*. Lining the canal of the

6

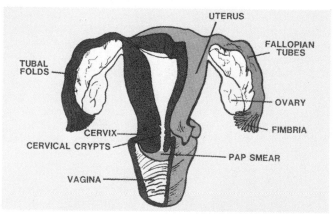

Fig. 2-4 A cut-away view of the uterus, fallopian tubes, ovaries, cervix, cervical crypts and vagina

cervix are the *cervical crypts*. It is within the cervical crypts that the cervical mucus is produced. The mucus is discharged to the outside of the woman's body where all of the observations in the Ovulation Method are made. There are no internal examinations involved in using the Ovulation Method. The location at the opening of the cervix where a *pap smear* is taken is also shown in Figure 2-4.

The menstrual cycle begins with the first day of menstrual bleeding and ends with the last day prior to the beginning of the next menstrual period. The length of this cycle tends to be somewhat irregular. While the average length of the menstrual cycle is around 28 days, most women will experience menstrual cycles from 21 through 38 or 40 days in duration during their reproductive life. Many people wonder why one menstrual cycle may be short while another may be more regular in length and still another may be long in duration.

In Figure 2-5, the phases of the menstrual cycle are shown. There are basically two phases that are important, the *preovulatory phase* and the *postovulatory phase*. The preovulatory phase of the cycle is counted from the first day of menstrual bleeding until the day of ovulation. The postovulatory phase of the cycle is counted from the day after ovulation until the day before the beginning of the next menstrual period.

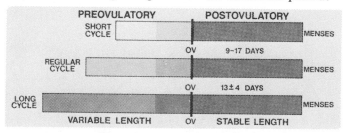

Fig. 2-5 The phases of the menstrual cycle

It is the preovulatory phase of the cycle which is highly variable. The postovulatory phase of the cycle is quite stable in its length. From the time of ovulation until the beginning of the next menstrual period averages about

13 days although a range of 9 to 17 days can be expected in a population of women. In the individual woman, however, there is great consistency in the length of the postovulatory phase of the cycle. It is the variable length of the preovulation phase which ultimately determines whether a cycle will be short or long.

If the preovulatory phase of the cycle was stable, then all one would have to do would be to calculate so many days from the first day of the menstrual cycle in order to determine one's fertility. However, the variability of this phase dictates against doing that. The Ovulation Method has finally allowed us to solve this problem. As can be seen by the lightly shaded areas which are present in the preovulatory phase of the three cycles in Figure 2-5, the mucus appears before ovulation and it gives advance indication that ovulation is approaching. As you learn the signs of ovulation which are associated with the cervical mucus observation, the information in this figure becomes highly practical. In fact, a woman will be able to predict the onset of her next menstrual period well in advance of its occurrence.

During the course of the menstrual cycle, there is a cyclic event occurring in the ovary called "the ovulation cycle" (Figure 2-6). The menstrual cycle and its accompanying ovulation cycle are the result of the close interaction of several hormones. The *pituitary gland* (the master gland of the body) is a small, pea sized gland which rests at the base of the brain. This gland produces two hormones which are very important to the smooth functioning of these cycles. They are called *FSH* and *LH*. The *FSH* stimulates the development of an egg in the ovary. The *LH* actually stimulates the release of the egg from the ovary.

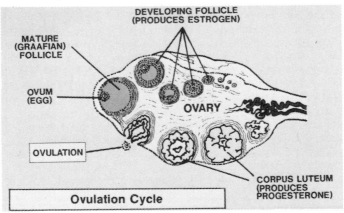

Fig. 2-6 The ovulation cycle

There are several hundred thousand individual, undeveloped eggs in the ovary. Early in the menstrual cycle, one or two of these eggs is selected to develop toward ovulation. These eggs develop within a *follicle*. A follicle is a small cyst-like structure. The follicle begins to grow and develop and just prior to ovulation is one inch or more in diameter. At that time it is called a mature follicle. With the rupture of this follicle, the egg is released from the ovary in a process called *ovulation*. The same tissue which was the mature follicle now becomes what is called a *corpus luteum*. That means, "yellow body" because it appears yellow on the ovary.

The developing follicle produces a hormone called *estrogen* which is the predominant preovulatory hormone and the one which stimulates the production of cervical mucus. After ovulation, the corpus luteum produces a hormone called *progesterone*. The progesterone hormone is the dominant postovulatory hormone. It stops the mucus production and is essential to the hormonal support to the lining cells of the uterus preparing them for pregnancy. Infertility or frequent spontaneous abortions (miscarriages) may be caused by an inadequate corpus luteum which does not produce enough progesterone.

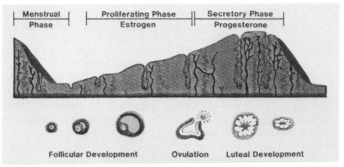

Fig. 2-7 The changes in the lining of the uterus

The changes which occur in the lining of the uterus during the course of the menstrual cycle are shown in Figure 2-7. It is the lining cells of the uterus which slough at the time of menstruation (Figure 2-8).

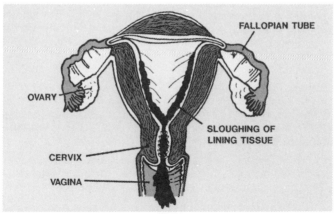

Fig. 2-8 Menstruation

With the sloughing of the lining cells of the uterus during the "menstrual phase" of the cycle, the lining of the uterus becomes very thin. Following menstruation, under the influence of the estrogen hormone, the lining cells of the uterus again begin to grow and develop in what is called the "proliferating phase" of the menstrual cycle. The ovulation cycle is also shown in Figure 2-7 to assist the reader in coordinating the events of the ovulation cycle with the events occurring in the lining of the uterus. The phase of follicular development coincides in the ovary with the proliferating phase in the lining of the uterus. Once ovulation has occurred and luteal development begins with the production of progesterone, the lining cells of the uterus begin to secrete a highly nutritious fluid. This is called the "secretory phase" of the menstrual cycle. It is during this phase of the cycle that im-

9

plantation of the new human life occurs following conception. If a pregnancy does not occur, the progesterone hormone level falls, removing its hormonal support to the lining of the uterus and the lining cells once again slough and a menstrual period occurs. The entire cyclic process then begins once again.

It is important to understand that ovulation occurs on only one day during a given menstrual cycle. Ovulation does not occur today and then again sometime next week. If this form of double ovulation did occur, of course, natural family planning would not work. This form of double ovulation is one of the old myths that needs to be dispelled when discussing natural family planning. Ovulation can, of course, occur twice or even three times in one cycle as non-identical twins and triplets would prove. However, when ovulation occurs twice in a menstrual cycle, it occurs within the same 24 hour time period. From a practical point of view, this form of double ovulation does not pose a problem for users of natural methods. As an addendum to this discussion, some people have felt that women ovulate in response to sexual stimulation. This is another myth which needs to be dispelled. The evidence for such sexually stimulated ovulation comes from experiments that have been performed in rabbits. Indeed, rabbits do ovulate in response to sexual stimulation, but humans do not.

Once ovulation occurs, the egg lives for only 12-24 hours if it is not fertilized. If anything, the life span of the egg is closer to 12 hours than it is to 24. This life span of the egg is so short that if our fertility depended upon this fact alone, few people would become pregnant during their entire reproductive life. But the length of the fertile period is extended by another *vital factor*. The vital factor is the cervical mucus. It is the cervical mucus which allows the sperm to survive long enough to become available when an egg is released and, of course, it is the cervical mucus that is involved in learning and understanding your fertility through the Ovulation Method.

The sperm need cervical mucus to survive. Sperm, in the absence of good mucus, will die literally within hours or even minutes when placed into the vagina. In the presence of good cervical mucus, however, the sperm may live from three to five days. Sperm survival is directly dependent upon the presence of good cervical mucus.

The hormone estrogen, to which reference has been made earlier, is extremely important in mucus production. This hormone reaches a very high level or a Peak approximately one day before ovulation.

The pattern of the two ovarian hormones, estrogen and progesterone, as they change throughout the menstrual cycle is shown in Figure 2-9. The first day of the menstrual cycle would be at the lower left hand corner of this graph and the last day of the menstrual cycle is at the lower right hand corner of the graph. The day of ovulation is shown by the vertical dotted line in the middle.

If you follow the estrogen curve, you will note that the estrogen level rises to a very high level, a Peak, just prior to the time of ovulation. It is this rise in the estrogen hormone which stimulates the production of the cervical mucus. After ovulation, the predominant hormone is progesterone. This hormone rises to very high levels following ovulation. The progesterone hormone inhibits the effects of the estrogen hormone on the production of cervical mucus. It also helps to prepare the lining cells of the uterus, as mentioned earlier, for the implantation of a new human life.

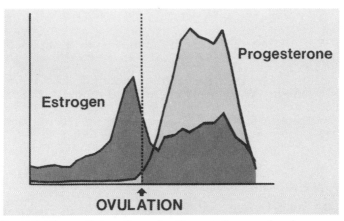

Fig. 2-9 The pattern of production of the ovarian hormones

A very important function of the cervical mucus in human fertility is shown in Figure 2-10. On the left side of the diagram is a very characteristic type of cervical mucus which is only produced when the estrogen levels are rising or are very high. This type of mucus arranges itself in *parallel strands,* forming, literally, swimming channels for the sperm so that they can penetrate through the cervix and go up to the fallopian tubes where conception will occur. This type of cervical mucus is called Type E mucus. On the right side is the type of mucus which is produced when the estrogen levels are very low or when the progesterone levels are high. This type of mucus is called Type G mucus and is very thick and dense and, in fact, acts as *a barrier to sperm penetration.*

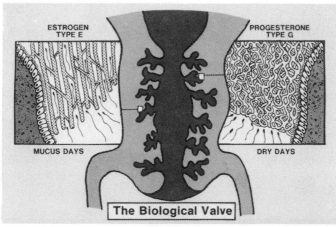

Fig. 2-10 The biological valve

These two types of cervical mucus act, in effect, like a *biological valve.* The valve is open, allowing sperm to penetrate through the cervix, when the Type E or estrogen stimulated mucus is present. The valve is closed to sperm penetration when the mucus is of the Type G variety. This biological valve is essential to human fertility and assures that fresh sperm and fresh eggs are available at the time of conception. In the Ovulation Method, the couple is

11

taught how to determine, in effect, when the biological valve is open and when it is closed.

Our fertility depends, then, on the presence of good sperm, good eggs and good cervical mucus. There are, of course, many other factors involved in the fertility process. However, the presence of good quality cervical mucus is nearly as important to the fertility process as the presence of good sperm and good eggs. We are only beginning to appreciate the role of cervical mucus as it relates to the overall reproductive process. However, when any one of these three factors is absent, the couple will not become pregnant.

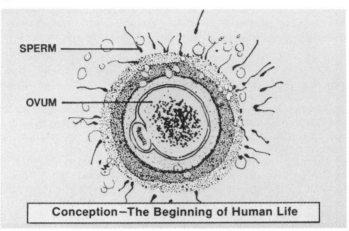

Conception—The Beginning of Human Life

Fig. 2-11 Conception - The Beginning of Human Life

When the sperm unites with the egg (ovum), a new human life comes into existence (Figure 2-11). This new life is different from any other that has ever existed. Each human life created in this fashion is unique and it is from this moment of conception that each of us began our life's journey.

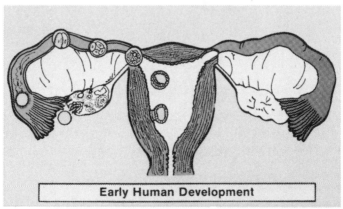

Early Human Development

Fig. 2-12 Early human development

Conception occurs in the outer portion of the fallopian tube (Figure 2-12). In the few days following *conception* the early process of human development continues with cell division. About six to nine days following conception, a process called *implantation* occurs. This is the process whereby the new human being nestles itself into the side wall of the uterus establishing its long term support system for its nine month journey toward birth.

The unborn child continues to grow and develop throughout the nine months within the uterus. The child at 16 weeks of age is shown in Figure 2-13. The placenta is in the upper left and the child is connected to that support system by his or her umbilical cord.

One final note for those who wish to use the Ovulation Method as a means of avoiding pregnancy. Pregnancy can result from *any genital contact* on days of fertility even without penetration or ejaculation. There is a fluid produced by the male with is called a *pre-ejaculatory fluid* and this fluid has a very high concentration of sperm. If that fluid (which can be pre-

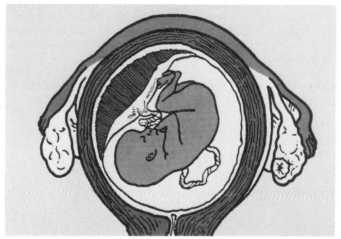

Fig. 2-13 The unborn child - 16 weeks of age

sent without ejaculation) comes into contact with the cervical mucus which is present at the opening of the vagina, the sperm can find their way to the fallopian tubes and a pregnancy can result. Therefore, a fundamental principal to the successful use of a natural method of family planning as a method to avoid pregnancy is the fact that it bases its effectiveness on the avoidance of all genital contact during the fertile time.

CHAPTER 3

MAKING GOOD MUCUS OBSERVATIONS

Research at the Creighton University Natural Family Planning Education and Research Center has resulted in a standardized system for making the observations of the cervical mucus discharge. This standardization is an important development in the Ovulation Method because it allows for a common system to be used by all users, provides for a common language in the use of the method, facilitates improvements in the method and allows for transfer of the client couple to a new teacher if they move throughout the country. In this chapter, this system will be explained. Such a system must become *routine* even if, on occassion, one part of the system may not reveal a pertinent observation. The *routine performance* of the observations assures that the mucus will be observed *when it is present*. This is a basic principle in making and using good mucus observations.

With this in mind, this system for observing the mucus, which has been thoroughly evaluated and tested in actual use, will now be presented.

THE THREE STEPS IN CHECKING THE MUCUS

There are essentially three steps in observing for the mucus. They are:

STEP 1—*Wipe the opening of the vagina* with toilet tissue paying attention to the *sensation* which this produces.

STEP 2—*Observe the tissue* for the presence or absence of mucus.

STEP 3—If mucus is present on the tissue, *finger test* the mucus between the thumb and index finger.

There are basically three components to making any one good mucus observation. The woman needs to determine the *sensation* that the mucus creates, she needs to determine its *stretchability and consistency* and to determine its *color*. The *basic principle* behind using three steps in checking for the mucus is in preventing any one part of making a good mucus observation to be either forgotten or ignored.

An easy way to remember the three steps is to remember the word **SOFT:**

S = **Sensation**
O = **Observation**
F = **Finger**
T = **Test**

It is *very important* to *make a decision* regarding the sensation the mucus creates when you are wiping with the tissue *prior to* looking at the tissue. The *sensation is extremely important*. It is something that the woman *feels*. It is *not* something she can see.

The second step in checking for the mucus is a *visual observation* of the tissue *to see* if mucus is or is not present. If mucus is present, then she moves to Step 3.

In the third step, mucus that is present on the tissue is lifted off and *finger tested* between the thumb and index finger. In this step, the stretchability of the mucus and its consistency is tested and the *color* of the mucus can be determined. *Whenever any mucus* is present on the tissue it *must* be finger tested. In addition, all areas of mucus that are present on the tissue *must* be finger tested. By finger testing all areas of mucus, errors in observing will be avoided.

When determining the color of the mucus this should be done only at the time of finger testing and then the mucus should be raised to *eye level* so that you can "look through" the mucus which is present.

HOW TO CHECK FOR THE MUCUS

A description is now provided on *how* to check for the mucus.

A. Use flat layers of tissue

B. Do not use crumpled tissue

In observing for the mucus, a few layers of *white,* non-scented, toilet tissue should be folded into a flat, rectangular shape of about 3 x 5 inches in dimension. This tissue is used to make the observation. Using flat layers of tissue makes the observation much easier. When crumpled tissue is used it is easy to "lose" the mucus in the creases of the tissue.

C. Wipe from front to back

D. Wipe from the urethra through the perineal body

In Figure 3-1, a diagram of the anatomy of the vulva is presented. It shows *where* the mucus should be observed. The wiping process should begin just in front of the urethra and proceed *between the labia, over the opening of the vagina,* through to the back portion of the vaginal opening half way over the *perineal body* toward the rectum.

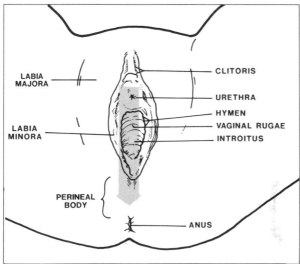

Fig. 3-1
A diagram of the vulvar anatomy. The arrow indicates the direction of observation for mucus and the area from the urethra through the perineal body which is wiped when observing mucus.

The mucus can be present at any place along this area. In addition, it has a tendency to collect near the back portion of the vagina just in front of the perineal body. Thus, wiping from the urethra through the perineal body is necessary so all of the mucus will be observed. In addition, wiping over the skin of the perineal body is important in a proper determination of the sensation. *The decision regarding the sensation should be made based upon the observation of the sensation as the tissue passes over the perineal body.*

16

E. Wipe until the mucus is gone

It is important that you wipe until the mucus is gone. It has been observed frequently that non-Peak type mucus is observed on the first wipe, only to observe Peak-type mucus on the second or even a third wipe. If the decision on the mucus observation is made only on one wipe then an important mucus observation can easily be missed. In addition, this instruction applies *at any time* the woman feels that a second wipe would be beneficial. Apparently the wiping process has the ability to "pull" mucus down toward the opening of the vagina. In effect, you should *wipe until dry*.

F. Do not do internal examinations

Internal examinations are *not* a part of the Ovulation Method. The method is based upon observing the mucus externally. Internal examinations create confusion and will provide misleading information for this method.

G. Do not check directly with the fingers

This standardized system of observing the mucus is based upon using toilet tissue to make the observations. Using fingers directly at the opening of the vagina will create confusion within this system.

H. Do not base the observations on what is observed in the underwear

It is not uncommon to see some discharge present on the underwear. However, the presence of this discharge does not generally correlate with the phases of fertility and infertility. Therefore, you should not base your observations on what is observed in the underwear. On occasion, an unusual observation may be observed in the underwear which may relate to your fertility. As one learns the Ovulation Method, one also learns good judgement relative to such observations.

WHEN TO CHECK FOR THE MUCUS

In addition to learning how to check for the mucus, the system continues in teaching the woman *when* to observe for the mucus.

A. Check every time you go to the bathroom

It is important that the mucus observation be made *every time* that you go to the bathroom. As a general rule, one does not have to make special trips to the bathroom to observe the mucus but when one goes to the bathroom an observation should be made. *This becomes part of your normal hygiene.* The important point here is that the mucus is *often seen only once during the day* and if you are not in the routine of observing every time you go to the bathroom, you can easily miss an important observation.

B. Check for the mucus every time before urination

C. Check for the mucus every time after urination

It is important in observing the mucus to observe both *before and after* urination. The mucus may be seen only before urination and not after and then again only after urination but not before. It cannot be predicted in advance when the mucus will be observed so, in order to make reliable observations, they should always be made both before and after urination.

D. Check for the mucus every time before a bowel movement

E. Check for the mucus every time after a bowel movement

It is important in observing the mucus to observe both *before and after* a bowel movement. The mucus may be seen only before a bowel movement and not after and then again only after a bowel movement but not before. It cannot be predicted in advance when the mucus will be observed so, in order to make reliable observations, they should always be made both before and after a bowel movement.

F. Check for the mucus every time before going to bed

G. Bear down every time before bed time

A last observation of the mucus should be made at the end of the day just prior to going to bed. Occassionally, this will be the only time that the mucus is present for the day and if an observation is not made at that time the mucus will be missed. The user should be aware that this observation should be made within 15 minutes of going to bed to go to sleep.

At this last observation prior to bedtime, you should also urinate and then bear down in a mild pushing similar to a bowel movement. This allows for any mucus which may be present to be pushed down where it can be observed by an external observation.

H. Make a decision at each observation

It is *extremely important* that you make a *definitive decision* regarding what has been observed *at the time* you make your observation. You should then make a *mental note* of that observation so that it can be recorded at the end of the day. This instruction becomes even more important as you become an experienced user of the method. Once the observations become *routine* the observations can be done so quickly that, unless a conscious decision is made at that time, the observation can be lost.

This process of making a mental note of the observation can be referred to as "registering" the observation. *Registering* is important if observations are not to be lost. In addition, the observation *must* be taken *as is*. There can be a tendency to *"negotiate"* an observation. The process of negotiating is the process whereby the actual observation is mentally "talked away" and replaced with a *false observation*. Usually, this occurs because one thinks that the actual observation just "couldn't be". Therefore, it is vitally important that you understand the importance of *registering and recording actual observations*.

I. Do not ever discontinue observations

In using the Ovulation Method, the observational routine must be adhered to 100% of the time. Therefore, discontinuing observations will make the method less effective.

J. Do not become complacent about making the observations

As you become more confident in the use of the method and the observations become easy for you, you need to be reminded that you should not become complacent or "lazy" in checking for the mucus. This will lead to poor observations and a poor record of your phases of fertility and infertility.

OBSERVATION OF THE MUCUS DURING MENSTRUATION

The menstrual period is a unique time for mucus observation. There are several important factors which need to be kept in mind. First of all, it is not unusual to observe a mucus-like discharge which occurs at the same time as the heavy days of menstruation and even, on occasion, on the moderate days. This mucus discharge comes from the lining of the uterus. As the menstrual period tapers and the flow becomes light and very light, the presence or absence of mucus is as easy to detect as if there were no menstrual period.

In using the Ovulation Method, we recommend that you use mini-pads during the light and very light days so that normal mucus observations can be made. Therefore, tampons should be avoided if at all possible. However, tampons can be used during the heavy and moderate days so long as they are changed frequently, at least every 4 to 6 hours and are not used during prolonged sleeping intervals.

SPECIAL TIMES TO CHECK FOR THE MUCUS

There are a few special times in checking for the mucus which the user of the Ovulation Method should be aware of. These are:

1. *When you get up at night to urinate.* Over 40% of women will get up at least once during the night to urinate. If you are one of those women, be sure to observe the mucus at that time.

2. *At the time of bathing or showering.* At the time of bathing or showering the mucus can be washed away when the vulva is washed. Therefore, you should observe for the mucus *prior to taking a bath or shower* and, as a general rule, *observe for the mucus whenever the vulva is wiped.*

3. *Before and after swimming.* Those women who swim have a unique concern regarding the mucus. Again, when toweling, the mucus may be wiped away. You should be aware of this possibility and observe for the mucus carefully before and after swimming.

THE EASE OF OBSERVING

The observational routine which has been described above is actually very easy to accomplish. In over 90% of women, this observational routine can be accomplished in 30 seconds or less.

GENERAL HYGIENE

The vagina is a self cleansing organ. *There is no need to douche.* Regular bathing is adequate for normal hygiene. Douching may actually wash away the mucus and is not to be done when using the Ovulation Method.

There are a number of toilet products which have perfumes in them. As a general rule, scented hygiene items should not be used. Those items which may contain such perfumes include tampons, pads, minipads, toilet tissue, fabric softeners, bubble bath, bath oils, etc. Indeed, even toilet tissue which is dyed can be irritating. The perfumes and the dyes can, in some women, stimulate a chemical irritation which resembles the symptoms of a vaginal infection. Only with discontinuation of the product do the symptoms disappear.

It is also preferred that women using the Ovulation Method wear underwear that is made of all cotton material or has a cotton crotch. Undergarments which are manufactured from synthetic materials repel moisture whereas cotton absorbs it. With the synthetic fibers, moisture tends to collect at the vulva and can be irritating, and, in some cases lead to confusion in making good mucus observations.

A FINAL NOTE

Making good mucus observations assists the woman and the couple in developing good feelings about themselves in the use of the method, developing their confidence and satisfaction. Checking accurately and knowing at the end of the day that the observations are correct can be helpful in your attitude toward the method.

CHAPTER 4

DESCRIBING THE MUCUS OBSERVATIONS

The previous chapter dealt with standardizing the observational routine. This chapter deals with standardizing the terminology which is used in describing the observations. When the information from the two chapters is put together, a standardized system for observing and recording the mucus observation evolves.

The following commentary is designed for use by *all* women. You may not observe everything that is described in this section, however, you will be able to select from this list *what you do observe*. This system has been developed through careful gynecologic evaluation of users of the Ovulation Method of natural family planning. Investigation has shown that women can relate extremely well to this system. It has been prepared with the generous assistance of the women who have helped us in our research.

WORDS THAT ARE USED IN DESCRIBING THE MUCUS

It is important that a common language be used in describing the mucus observations. With this in mind, the following definitions for words used in describing the mucus are provided:

Words Used To Describe "Stretchability"
Sticky = The mucus stretches up to ¼ inch
Tacky = The mucus stretches from ½ to ¾ inch
Stretchy = The mucus stretches *1 inch or more*

The words sticky, tacky and stretchy refer to the stretchability of the discharge. It is important to note that you do not need a ruler to make these determinations - you can easily estimate them.

Words To Describe Color
Clear = The mucus is crystal clear
Cloudy (White) = The mucus has a cloudy or white appearance to it. It may be opaque (that is, you can't see through it) or it may be translucent (somewhat "foggy" in its appearance).
Cloudy/Clear = The mucus is partly cloudy and partly clear. When this designation is utilized the clear means crystal clear.
Yellow = The mucus has a yellowish discoloration to it. This may indicate a small amount of blood present in the discharge or a low grade infection.
Red = This indicates that there is fresh blood in the discharge.
Brown = This indicates that there is old blood in the discharge.

Words Used To Describe Two Other Variations

There are two other types of discharge that a woman might observe while using the Ovulation Method. *These two types of discharge are very characteristic in their consistency.*

Pasty (Creamy) = **The pasty discharge is very similar to the consistency of flour paste or hand lotion. It may be sticky but it is *never* tacky or stretchy (by itself). It is usually cloudy or white in color, although on occasion it may be yellow.**

Gummy (Gluey) = **Some women may observe a very thick discharge which looks like half dried ariplane glue or rubber cement. It will often (but not always) have a yellowish discoloration to it. It may be sticky, tacky or stretchy.**

Words To Describe Sensations

A number of observations that a woman may make will not result in a discharge which can be finger tested. The observation of the mucus then *relies upon the sensation entirely.* This terminology is now explained and in the explanation we are using the "three steps" process for assisting you in understanding the observations. In addition, pictures of these observations along with all of the others described in this chapter, can be found in our publication *The Picture Dictionary of the Ovulation Method and Other Assorted Teaching Aids.*

Dry

1. When you wipe with this tissue you will feel the sensation of dryness. This will be a very *obvious* sensation.
2. As you observe the tissue you can see that it is dry and that it wrinkles easily.
3. Nothing can be finger tested from the tissue.
4. Dryness is generally not a problem for most women since it is such an *obvious* observation.

Damp *without* lubrication

Damp *with* lubrication

1. When you wipe with this tissue you *may* or *may not* observe a sensation of lubrication.
2. When you observe the tissue you will see an area of dampness on the tissue.
3. Nothing can be lifted off of this tissue to be finger tested.
4. The *key* to your fertility in this observation is the *presence* or *absence* of lubrication.
5. The observation of damp *without* lubrication has the same significance as a dry observation.
6. The observation of damp *with* lubrication is Peak-type mucus.

Shiny *without* lubrication

Shiny *with* lubrication

1. When you wipe with this tissue you *may* or *may not* observe the sensation of lubrication.
2. When you observe this tissue you will observe a damp area with small areas in the center which are shiny.

3. Nothing can be lifted off of this tissue to be finger tested.
4. The *key* to your fertility in this observation is the *presence* or *absence* of lubrication.
5. The observation of shiny *without* lubrication has the same significance as a dry observation.
6. The observation of shiny *with* lubrication is Peak-type mucus.

Wet *without* lubrication

Wet *with* lubrication

1. When you wipe with this tissue you *may* or *may not* observe a sensation of lubrication.
2. When you observe the tissue, the tissue is *very wet.* The wetness often has a glarey appearance to it which is different from the previous use of the term shiny.
3. Nothing can be lifted off this tissue to be finger tested.
4. The critical sign of your fertility in this observation, as with *damp* and *shiny,* is the *presence* or *absence* of lubrication.
5. The observation of wet *without* lubrication has the same significance as a dry observation.
6. The observation of wet *with* lubrication is Peak type mucus.

A NOTE ABOUT SENSATION

The sensation the mucus creates is *extremely important* to the proper use of the Ovulation Method. There are basically three sensations that a woman will observe: *dry, smooth and lubricative.* All three of these sensations are obvious. However, it is not unusual to confuse the smooth sensation for the lubricative one. This happens particularly in women who are not experiencing true lubrication and therefore think that the smoothness they feel is lubrication. Actually, the *dry and smooth* sensations belong to a broad category of *non-lubricative* sensations while lubrication is separate from those (Figure 4-1).

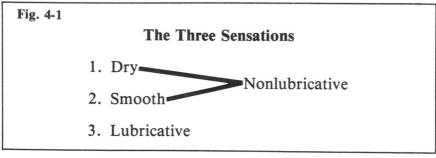

Fig. 4-1

The Three Sensations

1. Dry
2. Smooth — Nonlubricative
3. Lubricative

The decision regarding the sensation should be made at the time the woman wipes over the *perineal body.* In addition, she should make her decision regarding the sensation *prior* to looking at the tissue and finger testing the mucus. The sensations are *obvious ones.* When dryness is present she will feel definitely dry and the tissue will drag and develop a "scratchy" type of sensation. When the woman is lubricative the tissue will "glide" easily over the perineal body. When she has a smooth sensation, she will feel a smoothness as the tissue passes over the mucus membranes at the opening of the *vagina* but when the tissue passes over the perineal body it will have a "halting" tendency and move more roughly. That "halting" tells the woman that this is a smooth sensation, belonging to the non-lubricative categories, and that it is not true lubrication.

If after good observational technique there continues to be difficulty in observing the sensation, your teacher will be able to help you solve that problem. In concluding this chapter, the following reminders are provided:

1. Remember, you need only one of these three signs (clear, stretchy *or* lubricative) alone, or in any combination, to make the sign Peak-type mucus.

2. The word *sticky* refers to the stretch of the mucus up to ¼ *inch.*

3. The word *tacky* refers to the stretch of the mucus from ½ *to* ¾ *inch.*

4. The word *stretchy* refers to the stretch of the mucus *one inch or more.*

5. A ruler is not needed to make these observations.

6. Remember the special categories of *Peak-type mucus:* damp, shiny and wet *with* lubrication.

7. Remember the special categories of *"dry" observations:* damp, shiny and wet *without* lubrication.

8. In each of these latter observations, no mucus can be finger tested. Your fertility is determined by the sensation which is created during the wiping process.

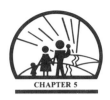

CHAPTER 5

CHARTING

Charting correctly the signs of fertility is very important to the successful use of the Ovulation Method. In addition, it is of great assistance to you in developing confidence. The chart is also an outstanding health record. This chapter outlines the basic principles of good charting.

DEFINITIONS
The following definitions are important during this discussion. You must know these definitions thoroughly in order to understand the instructions of the method.

> **Peak Type Mucus = Any mucus discharge that is clear, stretchy or lubricative. Any one of these three characteristics, alone or in any combination, results in the mucus discharge being defined as Peak type mucus.**
> **Non-Peak Type Mucus = Any mucus discharge that is not clear, stretchy, or lubricative. All three of these characteristics must be absent in order to establish the identity of non-Peak type mucus.**
> **The Peak Day = The last day of any mucus discharge that is clear, stretchy, or lubricative.**

THE BACK OF THE CHART
The back of the chart is shown in Figure 5-1. There is room for your name and a place for writing in the dates and times for each of the follow-up appointments.

In addition to the above bookkeeping items, a number of very important items are placed on the back of the chart. First of all, there is a section entitled *Definitions*. This section makes readily accessible the definitions of the terms Peak type mucus, non-Peak type mucus, and the Peak day. Secondly, the *Vaginal Discharge Recording System* is also on the back of the chart. This is for ready reference to assist the user in charting. Finally, an *instruction list* is provided so the teacher can provide specific instructions for you. The back of the chart is *extremely functional* and becomes an important focus in the learning process. The user should be fully aware of its contents so that it can be used readily.

NAME: ______ I.D. # ______ CHART # ______ TC ______ CC ______

NAME OF INSTRUCTOR: ______ TELE # ______

The Ovulation Method SHOULD NOT BE LEARNED without adequate instruction and follow-up from trained instructors. Make sure to come for your follow-up visits and refer any interested individuals for adequate instruction.

The Date Of Your Next Appointment	1	2	3	4	5	6	7	8

ALWAYS BRING YOUR CHART TO FOLLOW-UP

DEFINITIONS

PEAK TYPE MUCUS = Any mucus discharge that is CLEAR, STRETCHY, OR LUBRICATIVE.
NON-PEAK TYPE MUCUS = Any mucus discharge that is NOT clear, stretchy, OR lubricative.
THE PEAK DAY = The LAST DAY of any mucus discharge that is CLEAR, STRETCHY, OR LUBRICATIVE.

VAGINAL DISCHARGE RECORDING SYSTEM

H = Heavy flow	0 = Dry	B = Brown bleeding
M = Moderate flow	2 = Damp without lubrication	C = Cloudy (white)
L = Light flow	2W = Wet without lubrication	C/K = Cloudy/Clear
/L = Very light flow (spotting)	4 = Shiny without lubrication	G = Gummy (gluey)
	6 = Sticky (¼ inch)	K = Clear
Always record the presence or absence of mucus during the light and very light days of the menstrual flow.	8 = Tacky (½-¾ inch)	L = Lubricative
	10 = Stretchy (1 inch or more)	P = Pasty (creamy)
	10 DL = Damp WITH lubrication	Y = Yellow (even pale yellow)
	10 SL = Shiny WITH lubrication	
	10 WL = Wet WITH lubrication	

In addition, record how often during the day that you see the most fertile sign of the day and record it in the following fashion:
X1 = Seen only once that day X2 = Seen twice that day X3 = Seen three times that day AD = Seen All Day

INSTRUCTIONS

YOUR INSTRUCTIONS FOR USING THE METHOD WILL BE GIVEN TO YOU BY YOUR TEACHER, FROM THE LIST OF INSTRUCTIONS BELOW.

A. Always keep to the observational routine

B. Chart at the end of your day, every day, and record the most fertile sign of the day

C. Avoid genital contact

D. Days of fertility (use to achieve pregnancy)
1. The menstrual flow
2. From beginning of mucus until 3 full days past the PEAK
3. 1 or 2 days of NON-PEAK mucus PRE-PEAK
4. 3 or more days of NON-PEAK mucus PRE-PEAK – PLUS count 3
5. Any single day of PEAK mucus – PLUS count 3
6. Any unusual bleeding – PLUS count 3

E. Days of Infertility (use to avoid pregnancy)
1. Dry days pre-peak – end of the day, alternate days
2. Dry days pre-peak – end of the day, every day
3. 4th day post-peak – ALWAYS end of the day
4. Dry days post-peak (after 4th day) – end of the day, alternate days
5. Dry days post-peak (after 4th day) – end of the day, every day
6. Dry days post-peak (after 4th day) – anytime of the day
7. Dry days on L or VL days of bleeding at end of menstrual flow – end of the day

F. Seminal Fluid Instruction (see manual)

G. "Double" Peak
1. On P + 3 ask "double" peak questions
2. If post-peak phase greater than 16 days in duration and method used properly to avoid pregnancy, anticipate "missed" period form of "double" peak
3. When ANTICIPATING "DOUBLE" PEAK, keep to the end of the infertile days and continue good observations

H. When in doubt, consider yourself of peak fertility and count 3

I. Special Fertility Instructions
1. Avoid genital contact until good mucus is present (Subfertility patients only)
2. Use days of greatest quantity and quality and first two days afterward
3. Record the amount of stretch of the mucus (1", 2", 3" etc.), (subfertility patients only)
4. Record abdominal pain (AP), right abdominal pain (RAP), and left abdominal pain (LAP), (subfertility patients only)

J. Essential sameness question – "Is today essentially the same as yesterday?" – yes or no

K. Yellow Stamp Instructions
1. Pre-peak – end of the day, alternate days
2. Post-peak (after 4th day) – end of the day, alternate days
3. Post-peak (after 4th day) – end of the day, every day
4. Post-peak (after 4th day) – anytime of the day

L. If TOTALLY breastfeeding, first 56 days after birth of baby are infertile.

M. End of day instructions apply through the first normal menstrual cycle

N. Other (e.g. seminal fluid test, second wipe test, BBT, etc.)

NAME, ADDRESS AND TELEPHONE NUMBER OF NATURAL FAMILY PLANNING CENTER

Fig. 5-1 The back of the chart

THE INSIDE OF THE CHART

On the inside of the chart there are numbers across the top from 1 through 35. This tells the day of the menstrual cycle. For each day, there is a box provided for the placement of the proper stamp and another box provided for writing the proper description. In addition, there is a place provided to write in the date. The user should chart each new menstrual cycle beginning at the left margin of the chart and continuing it horizontally. There is room for six months of charting on each chart. The following could be considered the basic principles of good charting:

1. The client should begin charting immediately after receiving the initial instruction.

2. During the first month of charting or during the first complete cycle (whichever is shorter), the client should avoid genital contact so that the mucus can be seen in its natural state without being influenced by the presence of seminal fluid.

3. The client should chart the proper stamp and description at the end of each day during the cycle including the days of menstruation.

4. The client should chart the most fertile sign of the day.
5. The client should chart daily the "3 C'S" of the mucus.

        C = Consistency
        C = Color
        C = Change*
        S = Sensation

*The change is the day by day change in the consistency, color and sensation. Watching for obvious day by day changes is extremely important in understanding the nature of the mucus.

STAMPS

Stamps have been developed for use with the Ovulation Method. These stamps are used throughout the world.

Plain red stamps = For days of bleeding

Plain green stamps = For infertile dry days

White, baby stamps = For mucus days

Green, baby stamps = For dry days that are fertile (whithin the count of 3)

In addition to the above stamps, *yellow stamps* have also been used with use of the Ovulation Method. In this teaching system, yellow stamps should only be utilized upon specific indication and then only with the advice of the teacher.

DESCRIPTIONS

For each day of charting, a description is written in the description box. A standardized means for recording these has been developed and is discussed later in this chapter (see vaginal discharge recording system). In addition, the following signs are placed on the chart at the appropriate times:

P = Placed on a white, baby stamp on the Peak day.

1, 2, 3 = Placed on the three stamps following the Peak day.

I = An act of intercourse

The descriptions are extremely important. The user should record *the most fertile sign of the day* in the box provided. The Ovulation Method story is told in its day by day descriptions of the mucus patterns.

VAGINAL DISCHARGE RECORDING SYSTEM

The descriptions are the most important part of charting. They must accurately reflect the observations that the woman makes so that a true picture of the mucus patterns can evolve. The vaginal discharge recording system has been developed so that charting can be done more easily and its accuracy improved. You should use the *vaginal discharge recording system* from the very first follow-up. Experience has shown that it is very easy to learn and use and with its ready accessibility on the back of the chart you always have it for quick reference.

The recording system is outlined in Figure 5-2. While this recording system uses numbers, it should not be thought of as a scoring system. In effect, any form of symbolism could be used in the same fashion but a system of numbers and letters was chosen for this particular system. While there is a general tendency for the higher numbers to be associated with higher fertility, this should not be used in that way. The series of numbers and letters are simply a means of recording accurately the observations that you are making.

Vaginal Discharge Recording System

H = Heavy Flow	**0** = Dry	**B** = Brown Bleeding
M = Moderate Flow	**2** = Damp Without Lubrication	**C** = Cloudy (white)
L = Light Flow	**2W** = Wet Without Lubrication	**C/K** = Cloudy/Clear
VL = Very Light Flow (spotting)	**4** = Shiny Without Lubrication	**G** = Gummy (gluey)
	6 = Sticky (¼ inch)	**K** = Clear
Always record the	**8** = Tacky (½-¾ inch)	**L** = Lubricative
presence or absence	**10** = Stretchy (1 inch or more)	**P** = Pasty (creamy)
of mucus during the	**10DL** = Damp WITH Lubrication	**Y** = Yellow (even
light and very light days	**10SL** = Shiny WITH Lubrication	pale yellow)
of the menstrual flow.	**10WL** = Wet WITH Lubrication	

In addition, record how often during the day that you see the most fertile sign of the day and record it in the following fashion:

X1 = Seen only once that day	**X3** = Seen three times that day
X2 = Seen twice that day	**AD** = Seen All Day

Fig. 5-2 The vaginal discharge recording system

During the menstrual flow, the symbols H = heavy, M = moderate, L = light and VL = very light (or spotting) are used. *During the light and very light days of the menstrual flow an observation of the mucus should always be recorded.*

The numbers 0, 2, 2W and 4 all relate to observations which have the same significance as dry observations. In these cases, when you wonder what would be the "most fertile sign of the day", you would record the higher number. This is merely a convention for recording purposes and for accuracy of recording. All four of these recordings are thought of as dry observations relative to stamp placement and the use of the method instructions.

When the numbers 6, 8 and 10 are utilized, *a letter from the right hand column must always be utilized.* A color, consistency and/or sensation must be present when the mucus is stretchable.

The special categories of Peak type mucus are recorded as *10DL (damp with lubrication), 10SL (shiny with lubrication)* and *10WL (wet with lubrication).* Since in all of these observations lubrication is present and therefore the mucus is of the Peak type and would be of a high degree of fertility, the number 10 has been used in combination with the letters. The number 10 in this case does not mean stretchy. It is simply a means of recording these special categories of Peak type mucus.

In addition to the above recordings, it is also important to record how often during the day the most fertile sign of the day is observed. This is done by using X1 = seen only once that day; X2 = seen swice that day; X3 = seen three times that day; and AD = seen All Day. The latter designation means that the mucus has been observed four or more times during the day. Once it has been observed four times, you no longer need to keep a count of the number of times you have observed that most fertile sign. It automatically becomes an all day (AD) observation.

Examples of the Recording System in use:

1. Dry - Seen all day = 0 AD
2. Damp without lubrication - Seen all day = 2 AD
3. Stretchy, clear, lubricative - Seen all day = 10 KL AD
4. Sticky, cloudy - Seen only once = 6C X1
5. Tacky, gummy, yellow - Seen twice = 8 GY X2
6. Sticky, pasty, white - Seen twice = 6 PC X2

In the appendix, several charting examples are shown, all using the Vaginal Discharge Recording System.

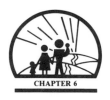

CHAPTER 6

BASIC METHOD INSTRUCTIONS

Understanding the instructions of the Ovulation Method is obviously fundamental to its proper use. The user couple must thoroughly know the instructions as they apply to different situations. This chapter is designed to provide a thorough grasp of these method instructions. It begins with a discussion of the basic principles.

BASIC PRINCIPLES

There are a number of basic principles which lay the foundation for the proper use of the method instructions. The couple should be thoroughly familar with these:

1. The Ovulation Method is a method of both achieving and avoiding pregnancy. It is not a method of contraception. It is a method of *true family planning.*

2. Users of the Ovulation Method are free to use the method to either achieve or avoid a pregnancy as they so choose.

3. It is the client couple's *responsibility* to *use* the method.

4. To achieve pregnancy the days of fertility are used.

5. To avoid pregnancy the days of infertility only are used.

6. Using days of fertility *abandons* the method as a method to avoid pregnancy and *adopts* the method as a method to achieve pregnancy.

7. There are no "taking chances" with the Ovulation Method. The method is either used as a method to achieve pregnancy or as a method to avoid pregnancy.

8. The method instructions include instructions regarding observations and charting, as well as the application of the instructions related to genital contact.

9. *The instructions related to genital contact evolve from one follow-up to the next* before the full method instructions are available to the user. This evolution of instructions is conducted under the supervision of the teacher.

10. The instructions related to genital contact *change* from one reproductive category to the next requiring additional teaching input at the time of a change in reproductive category.

11. The instructions to avoid pregnancy as they relate to observations, charting and genital contact have been developed so that, when used correctly, the method is over 99 percent effective as a method of avoiding pregnancy. *When the user chooses to deviate from these instructions they have chosen a less effective means to avoid pregnancy and have adopted a more effective means of achieving a pregnancy.*

DEFINITIONS

There are a number of definitions that are important for the couple to know so the instructions can be thoroughly understood. These definitions follow:

Peak-type mucus - Any mucus discharge that is clear, stretchy or lubricative.

Non-Peak type mucus - Any mucus discharge that is not clear, stretchy or lubricative.

The Peak day - The last day of any mucus discharge that is clear, stretchy or lubricative.

The pre-Peak phase - That phase of the menstrual cycle from the first day of menstruation up to and including the Peak day.

The post-Peak phase - That phase of the menstrual cycle from the day after the Peak day through the last day prior to the beginning of the next menstruation.

Genital contact - Any physical contact of the male and female genital organs. This includes the act of complete intercourse, an incomplete act of intercourse, close contact of the genital organs without intercourse, ejaculations within the vicinity of the female genital organs and any hand to genital contact. All genital contact must be avoided on the days of fertility if it is the intention to avoid pregnancy.

Sexual contact - Sexual contact is to be specifically distinguished from genital contact because it is the "contact" of the total person one to the other. Such contact includes genital contact but is much more than genital contact. In fact, most of the time, since it is a much broader concept, the physical act of intercourse is not involved. Sexual contact involves true sexual interaction and is therefore multi-dimensional. It is creative, intellectual, emotional, spiritual and physical. While genital contact is to be avoided during the days of fertility if it is the intention to avoid pregnancy, *sexual contact is never to be avoided.*

Unusual bleeding - Bleeding which is interpreted by the woman as being any bleeding other than a normal (usual) menstrual flow.

Variable return of Peak-type mucus - This refers to a condition in which the Peak-type mucus tends to come and go due to rising and falling levels of estrogen. It is most commonly observed in the *breastfeeding* woman who is in the weaning process and in women who are either *anovulatory or oligoovulatory.*

End of the day - The end of the day is considered to be that time of the day when the woman goes to bed to go to sleep.

Alternate days - Alternate days refers to every other day. In the instructions related to genital contact, this instruction recommends genital intercourse on one day, a day is then skipped where no genital contact occurs and then, on the next day, genital intercourse may be resumed.

Mucus patch - A series of one or more consecutive days of non-Peak type mucus unassociated with any Peak type mucus.

Contact pregnancy - Any pregnancy which occurs as the result of genital contact excluding the complete act of genital intercourse.

A NOTE ON THE PEAK DAY

The Peak day is the *last day* of any mucus which is clear, stretchy or lubricative. The Peak day is, obviously, determined one or two days after it

occurs. One of the most important factors which goes into identification of the Peak day is the *abrupt and dramatic* change in the pattern of the mucus which occurs after it. This abrupt change in the mucus pattern is due to the effects of the progesterone hormone, which rises after ovulation, on the production of cervical mucus. Women can very easily identify the last day of Peak type mucus and this abrupt or dramatic change which occurs in the days that follow. When these changes occur and one or two cycles pass which *confirm the woman's observations with the presence of menstruation following at the appropriate time,* the woman will establish *her confidence* in the identification of the Peak day. Using the instructions of the method which apply to the post-Peak phase of the cycle *requires confident identification of the Peak.* Development of confidence in this observation generally takes only one or two cycles.

It must be kept in mind that the identification of the Peak day is *not* based upon the *amount of the mucus.* The Peak day is the *last day of any* mucus that is clear, stretchy or lubricative. This means that *any one of these three signs, alone, or in any combination or amount* determines the presence of Peak type mucus. Not infrequently the amount of mucus might be relatively small but the characteristics of the mucus are still present allowing for a proper identification of Peak type mucus and the Peak day. Of all the clinical signs currently available for the detection of ovulation, the Peak day is the most accurate and reproducible.

In certain situations, especially the breastfeeding-weaning category and in women who are anovulatory, the woman will experience *a variable return of Peak type mucus.* In a situation such as this, the woman may experience several different days which fit the definition of "the last day of any mucus which is clear, stretchy or lubricative". In situations such as this, ovulation, if it occurs at all, is associated with the last Peak day. This last Peak day should be referred to as *the* Peak day. All of the other "Peak days" should be referred to as *a* Peak day. Having *"a* Peak day" simply allows conveyance of the message that Peak type mucus was present but thought not to be associated with ovulation. Having "the Peak day" implies that the buildup of the mucus and the abrupt change following the Peak day was typical of that associated with ovulation. This has practical importance in charting and in knowing and understanding the instructions. In the early months of learning, a "P" should be placed on any Peak day. It is optional, however, in later charting, to put a "P" on "a Peak day", whereas, a "P" should always be placed on "the Peak day". In addition it is necessary for "the Peak day" to have passed in order for the instructions which apply to the post-Peak phase of the cycle to be applicable. If only "a Peak day" has passed, the user continues to be pre-Peak and the pre-Peak instructions continue to apply.

BASIC METHOD INSTRUCTIONS

In most situations where the Ovulation Method is used there is a set of *basic instructions* which apply. While there are times, especially related to specific reproductive categories, where *special instructions* apply temporarily prior to instituting the basic instructions *it is the basic instructions which are the foundation of the method.* The following discussion explains the basic instructions (A charting example of the Basic Method Instructions can be found in Figure A-1 of the Appendix).

A. Always keep to the observational routine

It is important to realize that making *100 percent observations* in accordance with the routine previously discussed is an instruction of the method.

One's ability to define the time of fertility and infertility depends upon the adequacy of the observations that are made. This instruction is as important for those who wish to use the method to achieve a pregnancy as it is for those who wish to avoid a pregnancy. There is a tendency when using the method to achieve a pregnancy to eliminate some of the observations. This is a throwback to the contraceptive idea that in order to achieve a pregnancy one has to "stop the method". When using the Ovulation Method, good observations should be used and encouraged whichever way the method is being used.

B. Chart at the end of your day, every day, and record the most fertile sign of the day.

Charting should begin *immediately* (no later than the next day) after the Introductory Session. It, too, should be viewed as an extremely important element in the successful use of the method. It should also be kept in mind that the Ovulation Method chart is an *excellent health record.*

Charting should be done at the *end of the day* and the chart should be kept in a convenient location which is readily accessible to *both* the husband and the wife. Charting can be done by *either spouse.* Good charting habits include charting *every day* and not leaving several days at a time to chart. One's recollection of observations decreases proportionately with the time which transpires after the observations are made. And finally, the charting requires only the recording of the *most fertile sign of the day.* A record of every specific observation is unnecessary and not recommended.

C. Avoid genital contact

The initial instruction regarding the use of the method provided at the time of the introductory session is for the couple to avoid genital contact for either one month or one cycle, whichever is shorter. This instruction allows them an opportunity to observe the mucus discharge without confusion from seminal fluid. This instruction is *extremely important* to the development of *confidence* in the observations. There are *no exceptions* to it. Those couples who choose to have intercourse during this time should anticipate delays in learning and the development of confidence, as well as, a higher pregnancy rate.

Special instructions regarding the avoidance of genital contact apply to the infertility couple and to totally breastfeeding (see Appendix).

DAYS OF FERTILITY
(USED TO ACHIEVE PREGNANCY)

Usually at the second follow-up, the days of fertility and infertility are explained. The days of fertility are those days which, if used, the potential for pregnancy exists. The user couple should expect to become pregnant when these days are used.

A. The menstural flow

The menstrual flow is considered fertile for two reasons. First of all, every woman will experience a *short menstrual cycle* as the result of an *early ovulation* sometime during her reproductive life. When this happens, the beginning of mucus occurs during the tail end days of the menstrual flow and ovulation follows shortly thereafter. In this situation, intercourse during this time could result in a pregnancy. The second reason for considering the menstrual period fertile is the possibility of confusing a true menstrual period with bleeding that occasionally occurs at the time of ovulation (so called *"ovulation bleeding"*). In a small percentage of women, bleeding will occur around the time of ovulation as the result of the hormonal changes occurring at that time. This bleeding, of course, would be occurring at a time of Peak fertility. If bleeding were thought to be infertile and intercourse occurred on those days, a pregnancy would be expected to result.

Some degree of modification of this instruction has been developed (see below). When this modification is instituted, it takes precedence, for the light and very light days of menstrual bleeding.

B. From the beginning of the mucus until three full days past the Peak day

Fertility starts at the beginning of the mucus discharge and is present each day that the mucus is present as it builds up to the Peak day. Fertility continues through three full days past Peak day (infertility begins at the end of the fourth day). This instruction applies whether it is *a* Peak day or *the* Peak day.

C. Any one or two days of non-Peak mucus pre-Peak

The Ovulation Method is a *prospective* method by which the time of fertility can be identified. The method does not rely upon past cycles or previous calculations. When one or two days of non-Peak mucus appears, pre-Peak, it is judged to be fertile because it could be the beginning of the mucus buildup to the Peak day. If there is one day or two consecutive days of non-Peak mucus during the pre-Peak phase of the cycle and dry days follow this pattern, experience has shown that these dry days are infertile.

One is considered *to be pre-Peak* until one has *confidently identified the Peak day.*

D. When there are three or more days of non-Peak mucus pre-Peak, these days are fertile plus an additional three full days

When three or more consecutive days of non-Peak mucus occur during the pre-Peak phase of the cycle, the possibility that ovulation has been associated with this pattern increases and a count of three days follows the *last day* in which the non-Peak mucus occurs. It should be noted here that if, for example, there are three days of non-Peak mucus, a dry day and then three additional days of non-Peak mucus, the second three day mucus patch should be considered separately. Thus, the count of three starts on the dry day, but is interrupted by the second non-Peak mucus patch and a second three day count must follow the last day of the second three day mucus patch.

E. Any single day of Peak-type mucus is fertile plus an additional count of three days

When the mucus is of the Peak type, only one day of mucus is necessary to stimulate a count of three days. That one day would be considered fertile as would the next three days. This applies whether the woman is pre or post-Peak unless she is on special instructions for post-Peak mucus of this type.

F. Any unusual bleeding is considered fertile plus an additional three days

Bleeding which is thought to be other than a normal menstrual period *(unusual bleeding)* is considered in this method to be of Peak fertility and an additional three days of fertility should be added after the last day of unusual bleeding. In addition, to the best of the user's ability, whatever mucus discharge is observed or not observed during this unusual bleeding episode should also be recorded. The reason that unusual bleeding is considered fertile is because of the occasional association of such bleeding with ovulation.

The identification of *unusual bleeding is left to the woman's discretion* and is identified with specific reference to a normal menstrual period. The menstrual period has typical flow characteristics to it which a woman quickly learns to identify. Bleeding that is other than the normal menstrual period is different and is easily distinguished by the woman.

DAYS OF INFERTILITY
(USED TO AVOID PREGNANCY)

The following days are used if it is the couple's intention to use the Ovulation Method as a means of avoiding pregnancy. These instructions can be considered to be highly reliable indicators of infertility.

A. Dry days pre-Peak - end of the day, alternate days

The dry days during the pre-Peak phase of the cycle are considered infertile (if they are not within a count of three) because they are an indication that the ovary has not yet begun its progression toward ovulation. The infertility of the pre-Peak dry days, however, is *always* an *end of the day* instruction. It is necessary for the woman to observe the mucus throughout the entire course of the day to be certain of the infertility of that day.

In the early phases of learning, the couple is also instructed to use *alternate days*. This instruction allows them to gain confidence in their understanding of the seminal fluid. This means the utilization of the seminal fluid instruction with elimination of the seminal fluid discharge the day following intercourse. However, if a discharge is observed the day following intercourse it should be observed on its merits as a discharge (see Appendix). The alternate days instruction is temporary, usually only lasting the first one or two cycles of use and is specifically designed to assist the woman in gaining confidence in her observations without making errors in the early days of learning.

B. Dry days pre-Peak - end of the day, every day

Once the woman develops confidence in the use of the seminal fluid instruction and the day following intercourse is consistently dry (see discussion on seminal fluid instruction, Appendix) then the couple can move to an every day instruction. Intercourse can occur during each of the pre-Peak dry days at the end of the day with this instruction.

With pre-Peak dry days, the couple should be aware that the use of any other time of the day than the end of the day is to use the method in a less effective means as a method to avoid pregnancy and a more effective means as a method of achieving pregnancy. Having morning, afternoon, early evening or middle of the night intercourse during these days should be considered *achieving related behavior* since the pregnancy rate will be higher (see chapter 7).

C. Fourth day post-Peak - always end of the day

Infertility begins after the Peak day on the fourth day post-Peak *always at the end of the day*. This instruction allows an adequate time for the ovum to disintegrate so that infertility is indeed present.

D. Dry days post-Peak (after the fourth day) - end of the day, alternate days

The dry days during the post-Peak phase of the cycle, after the fourth day, are considered to be infertile. In the initial learning stages, because the woman needs to develop confidence in her identification of the Peak day, an essentially pre-Peak instruction is continued throughout the cycle (including post-Peak).

E. Dry days post-Peak (after fourth day) - end of the day, every day

As learning progresses and understanding of the seminal fluid advances, the couple can quickly progress to an end of the day, every day instruction. This means that all of the dry days during the post-Peak phase of the cycle are to be considered infertile (excluding the three day count) for an end of the day act of intercourse. This instruction is to be considered an interim, temporary instruction as the couple develops an understanding of the seminal fluid and confidence in the Peak day. In the occasional woman who cannot develop confidence in the Peak day, this instruction will be continued until such confidence develops.

F. Dry days post-Peak (after fourth day) - anytime of the day

Once the woman has developed *confidence* in her identification of the Peak day, the couple can then be moved onto an instruction which allows intercourse anytime of the day after the fourth day post-Peak. Such an instruction is based upon the concept that once the Peak day has passed so too has ovulation.

G. Dry days on the light and very light days of bleeding at the end of the menstrual flow - end of the day

When the woman has entered into the light and very light days of the menstrual flow, she can identify with confidence after a short period of time the presence or absence of mucus on those days. Those days can then be utilized in the same fashion as any other pre-Peak days. If the days have mucus, that would define days of fertility. If the days are dry, intercourse should occur at the end of the day.

This instruction should not be implemented until at least three menstrual flows have been consistently, accurately and confidently charted.

H. "Double" Peak

Instructions related to a "double" Peak should be considered a basic method instruction (see Appendix).

I. When in doubt, consider yourself of Peak fertility and count three

Whenever the couple has doubt in regard to the use of the method, they should consider themselves of Peak fertility during the time of the doubtful period and count three days of additional fertility following the single day or last day of doubt. This is an important instruction which covers any unusual happening which may create confusion in the couple's minds. Perhaps observations have been missed or forgotten; perhaps an unusual set of circumstances occurs which creates confusion. When such doubt exists, and it is your intention to avoid pregnancy,you should consider that time Peak fertility. In addition, when such confusion exists, you should contact your natural family planning teacher or natural family planning center so that the questions you have can be answered and the doubt can be relieved. This instruction is more important than it would initially appear. Every couple will be in a situation such as this occasionally.

ACHIEVING PREGNANCY

In Figure A-2 of the Appendix, the use of the Ovulation Method to achieve a pregnancy in a couple of normal fertility is demonstrated. As a general rule when a couple utilizes the days of Peak fertility, the chances they will achieve a pregnancy are extremely high. While definitive data is not yet available, a preliminary survey of 50 pregnancies indicated that over 75 percent of the couples (of normal fertility) became pregnant in the very first cycle in which they utilized the days of fertility.

While the days of fertility which are listed in the basic method instructions have been developed to provide a method which is highly reliable to avoid pregnancy, some of the instructions are less effective when actually used to achieve a pregnancy. Thus, a special fertility instruction has been developed. It is:

A. Use days of greatest quantity and quality and first two days afterward

This instruction has been developed upon a common sense assertion that these would be the days of highest fertility during the course of a menstrual cycle. However, it should be made clear that, at the present time, there is no organized set of data which specifically proves this instruction. Nonetheless, experience shows that an instruction such as this is worthwhile in assisting the couple to focus their efforts in achieving pregnancy at this particular time of the cycle. Caution should be exercised, however, for those couples who are using the method to avoid pregnancy. They must not be led to believe that some of the days which are listed previously as days of fertility can now be observed as infertile. *If that assumption is made then the effectiveness of the method will be lowered considerably as a means of avoiding pregnancy.* This special fertility instruction is designed only to augment the method's effectiveness as a means of achieving pregnancy.

CHAPTER 7

LEARNING S-P-I-C-E

The use of any method of natural family planning requires the adoption of a form of behavior which, if it is the couple's intention to avoid pregnancy, requires that genital contact be periodically avoided. Often, this is thought of as a "side effect" or "complication" of the method. In actual fact, it is probably the most important behavioral component in the use of a natural method since it allows the couple to place into proper perspective the totality of their human sexuality. While we live in a society whose sexual ethos is genitocentric, it is the great challenge of the natural family planning user to understand and appreciate the cerebrocentric nature of their human sexuality. It is with this in mind that the concept of sexual contact is distinguished from the concept of genital contact.

Genital contact is any physical contact of the male and female genital organs. This includes the act of complete intercourse, an incomplete act of intercourse, close contact of the genital organs without intercourse, ejaculations within the vicinity of the female genital organs and any hand to genital contact. All genital contact must be avoided on the days of fertility if it is the intention to avoid a pregnancy. From that perspective, the avoidance of genital contact is the primary mechanism through which the Ovulation Method works in avoiding pregnancy.

Sexual contact is to be specifically distinguished from genital contact because it is the "contact" of the total person one to the other. Such contact includes genital contact but is much more than genital contact. In fact, most of the time, since it is a much broader concept, the physical act of intercourse is not involved. Sexual contact involves true sexual interaction and is therefore multidimensional. It is spiritual, physical, intellectual, creative and emotional (S-P-I-C-E). While genital contact is to be avoided during the days of fertility if it is the intention to avoid pregnancy, *sexual contact is never to be avoided*.

By avoiding genital contact on a periodic basis, there is a natural tendency for the couple to communicate in other, non-genital ways. Such communication really forms the foundation for a joyful and lasting marriage relationship. When genital contact becomes the primary focus of the relationship, the communicative aspects of one's personality are left undeveloped. Trust in a relationship comes from the development of non-genital forms of communication. With this, a true communion between man and woman can develop which is liberating, loving and permanent. In addition, when such love exists, the genital union takes on a deeper meaning and its quality is elevated.

LEARNING S-P-I-C-E

Couples can modify their genital behavior without a great deal of difficulty if they desire to do so. To have genital intercourse is not an uncontrollable urge. However, learning to relate in a non-genital way is a big

39

challenge for the couples who enter a natural family planning program especially those who have a long history of contraceptive use. The important factor for them is the development of all aspects of their relationship so that a balance and perspective is allowed to enter into their lives.

The user of natural family planning will be involved in developing *new patterns of sexual interaction.* These new patterns are usually in the nongenital areas of human sexuality. We call this *LEARNING S-P-I-C-E. S-P-I-C-E refers to the development of the multidimensional nature of true sexual interaction.* This involves the development of the Spiritual, Physical, Intellectual, Creative/Communicative, Emotional/Psychological (SPICE) aspects of your sexuality. This can be assisted by reviewing some concrete examples of nongenital forms of sexual interaction.

From this perspective, for each of the components of S-P-I-C-E, a list of concrete suggestions which the user may reflect on is now presented. The couple should realize that this listing is far from complete but we offer it in the hope that it will stimulate further development of these areas.

Spiritual

1. Perhaps the most significant spiritual conponent of nongenital sexual interaction is *prayer.* Prayer is an essential component to the development and strengthening of the spiritual needs of the individual and the couple.

2. If the couple can be brought to the knowledge that their ultimate love is for God and that the love for one's spouse evolves from this then an enormously important foundation is provided for the activities of natural family planning.

3. Verbally communicating to the spouse that "I love you and I love everything about you" is a profoundly spiritual (as well as emotional and psychological) experience. As this is reiterated in daily life it assists in the development of a trust which cannot be shaken.

Physical

1. Couples should not sleep in separate bedrooms. Couples should sleep together, as they normally do, during the time when they are avoiding genital contact.

2. The "honeymoon effect" is well known in natural family planning. As the couple avoids genital contact during the time of fertility, the onset of the infertile time creates a very special quality to the act of genital intercourse.

3. Nonorgasmic touching and embracing should be encouraged among couples using natural family planning. Hugging, kissing, holding hands or just being held can be powerful experiences. Perhaps one of the best kept secrets is that men like to be held as do women.

4. "Creative cuddling" is a means of physically expressing ones closeness without leading to genital intercourse. One of the exciting experiences of natural family planning is falling asleep in each others arms without any demands being placed on either spouse. It is often important for the couple to discuss their individual "fine-lines" beyond which genital arousal is experienced. By openly discussing these, each spouse can fully respect the other.

5. The period of time in which the couple avoids genital contact is often experienced by the couple as "a break" from needing to "perform" every night.

6. An important form of physical activity involves the spouse' physical relationship with his/her children. Playing with the children, hugging and kissing them, and generally reinforcing their security, is a means of truly being life giving to them in an ongoing way. Such an important form of interaction also seems to reduce the need for genital activity. It does this by increasing the self-esteem of the father or mother.

7. A variety of other physical activities can also be engaged in such as going for walks, setting up special times to talk and plan the days ahead, watching a late movie together, etc. These activities are bridge building and communication stimulating. Again, they build trust in a relationship and increase the self estem of the couples thereby reducing the need for its superficial reinforcement with genital intercourse.

Intellectual
1. Reading materials can often be used to assist in broadening these concepts.

2. Understanding how natural family planning is respectful of our bodies and ourselves can intellectually be supportive to the use of natural family planning and the decisions to avoid genital contact.

3. The couple should discuss their priorities with regard to the use of the method. Do they wish another child at this time? If not, why not? Verbal discussion on their intentions in using the method are very important to developing a positive attitude toward genital avoidance.

Creative/Communicative
1. One of the spouses could make something special for the other, perhaps a special meal or a quiet dinner together. A husband's bringing flowers to his wife or doing other special things which he knows she will appreciate helps build a communion between husband and wife. Some couples write love letters to each other finding that writing how they feel is a special means of communicating one to the other. A wife may put a special note in her husbands lunch box saying "I love you" or the husband may call home during the day and simply say "Hi, how are you? I love you."

2. Doing projects together, organizing them and planning for them creates the opportunity for jointly working together. Projects around the home, planting a garden, family outings are examples of this type of activity.

3. You can individually make a list of ten special, nongenital ways of loving which would be meaningful and then exchange the two lists so that you can mutually discuss and learn from them. Such an activity can assist the couple in formulating in a creative way, those features of nongenital sexual interaction which are unique to them.

Emotional/Psychological
1. The couple should reserve special time for themselves so they can talk about their day or other things which would be of importance to them.

2. Couples should explore and express their feelings. While the expression of their needs and feelings may be new for them they should be encouraged and supported in their efforts. Such endeavors, done within the context of trust can be very important to developing openness within the relationship.

3. Couples should be allowed to ventilate their frustrations and know that such frustrations are normal. How do you feel about avoiding genital contact? You can discuss these questions together and learn from each other.

Through this process of ventilating frustration and even anger, the couple can begin to recognize important concerns of the other. With this process, resolution of the difficulties can be worked through. It is important, however, that *resolution* take place since the simple expression of frustration or anger is incomplete by itself.

4. Couples should be totally open in their relationship. As the relationship "opens up" there is a *bonding* which occurs in the relationship and the feelings of closeness and intimacy become profound. Genital contact is not a requirement for this bonding.

5. Finally, the couple should have a *sense of humor.* Being able to laugh at oneself and at each other at the appropriate time is an important release for couples.

Natural family planning is unique in its ability to stimulate new, nongenital forms of sexual interaction. The full excitement of using natural family planning comes only if couples venture into these new areas and experience S-P-I-C-E.

ACHIEVING AND AVOIDING RELATED BEHAVIOR

The Ovulation Method can be used to either achieve or avoid pregnancy. This is a use-related concept which is unique to natural family planning. It is this feature which truly distinguishes these methods from methods of contraception. In actual fact, natural methods are the only ones whose use does not have to be discontinued in order to become pregnant.

Obviously, if the couple is utilizing the method according to its instructions as a method to avoid a pregnancy, they are exhibiting *avoiding related behavior.* At the same time, if a couple turns around and knowingly uses days of peak fertility, this is clearly *achieving related behavior.* These two examples would be reasonably obvious to most people. The challenge in natural family planning is to understand the more subtle aspects of avoiding and achieving related behavior.

The days of fertility as defined by the Ovulation Method are very precise. In fact, they are so precise that they have the potential of revolutionizing our approach to the whole concept of achieving a pregnancy. There is no such thing as "taking a chance" when using the Ovulation Method. In fact, the Ovulation Method makes archaic that notion which grew up with the Calendar Rhythm Method. *In actual fact, "taking a chance" is the use of days which carry with them a higher pregnancy rate.* Thus, such behavior properly belongs within the classification of achieving related behavior.

It is relatively easy to identify avoiding related behavior; *the observations are followed 100 percent, the charting is accurately accomplished and the instructions to avoid a pregnancy are followed perfectly.* If the method is used in that fashion, it can be anticipated to be highly reliable in avoiding pregnancy. Any deviation from the basic instructions to avoid a pregnancy should be expected to lower the effectiveness of the method as a method of avoiding pregnancy. Actually, by lowering the effectiveness to avoid pregnancy, these deviations increase the method's effectiveness to achieve a pregnancy. *Thus, whenever actions are taken which increase the pregnancy rate those actions can be defined as achieving related behavior.*

Some specific achieving related behavior can be identified. For example, when a woman begins to drop observations even though she is fully cognizant of the importance of those observations or when a couple uses beginning of the day intercourse during the pre-peak phase of the cycle when they know that the instruction is for the end of the day; or when the couple uses the third day post-peak thinking that they "most likely" won't become pregnant - these are forms of *achieving related behavior*. Even when a couple is in a state of *ambivalance* regarding their intentions on how to use the method they are in an achieving related state. Once the couple has deviated away from the decision to avoid a pregnancy and, even though they have not reached a full conscious level of deciding to achieve a pregnancy, their move away from avoiding related intention is a form of achieving related behavior.

It is important for the couple to realize that the achieving related behavior often runs ahead of "full scale" achieving related intention. Not to decide is to decide.

As our understanding of our fertility increases, the potential exists for couples to engage in truly conceptional acts. Rather than "sneak up" on a pregnancy, the couple can reach a level of being able to consciously co-create with God a new human life.

DECISION MAKING IN THE USE OF THE OVULATION METHOD

One of the important facts in a mature use of the Ovulation Method is an understanding within the couple of how decision making occurs while using the method. In our society, we have all grown up with the notion that the basic decision is "Should we or should we not have intercourse?" However, in natural family planning, the decision is "Should we or should we not have another child?"

This is an extremely important principle for putting into right focus the approach to decision making in the use of the Ovulation Method. It is important for couples to learn this reality which is at the base of their decision making. It is completely different in its perspective than contraceptive use.

For a couple using the Ovulation Method of natural family planning, the ultimate decision on whether or not to have genital intercourse at a particular time revolves around whether or not their intentions in using the method are to achieve or avoid a pregnancy. If it is the couple's intention to avoid a pregnancy and it is a time of fertility it is a *sine que non* for the proper use of the method (to avoid pregnancy) not to have genital intercourse at that time. Thus, communication with regard to the utilization of certain days of the cycle should revolve around the couple's discussion of their intentions on how they wish to use the method not whether or not they should have genital intercourse at that time. That is a secondary decision. Once the primary decision is settled then the question of genital intercourse is also settled. However, if one focuses only on the decision to have genital intercourse as the primary decision making process, errors can easily be made in the couple's intention-specific use of the method. In addition, that approach is not realistic in the use of a natural family planning method.

When a couple is deciding whether or not to have intercourse, it is not uncommon for the husband to ask "Can we have intercourse tonight?" This puts his wife into the awkward position of being the "broker" who must say "yes" or "no." To alleviate this problem, the couple should look at their chart together and determine first if the day is a day of fertility or infertility and if it is a day of fertility, discuss the question "Do we wish to have a child at this time?" If the answer is yes to that question then the answer could be yes to having genital intercourse. However, if the answer is no to that question then the answer is no to genital intercourse. In this way, the couple is entering into the joint communication which is vital to the mature use of the Ovulation Method.

BASIC BEHAVIORAL ISSUES

1. *Difficulty in avoiding genital contact.* It is important not to assume that all couples will deal with avoiding genital contact in a positive way. Clarification as to which partner is having the difficulty in maintaining genital avoidance is also important since there is a tendency to assume that it is automatically the male when, in fact, it may be the female who is having the most difficulty. In addition, it is important to clarify what you hope to gain from having genital intercourse. Perhaps you view genital intercourse as the only or the primary way of expressing closeness. If this is true, you can be helped in understanding that an expanded fulfillment can come from a feeling of being understood and accepted, from sharing and from closeness, rather than just performing an act together. Learning S-P-I-C-E is involved with this basic behavioral issue.

It is not "wrong" to have the desire for genital intercourse at the time of fertility; but these feelings do not necessarily have to end in intercourse. They can be very adequately satisfied in other nongenital ways. If you have these feelings, however, learn to express them to one another and not to keep them inside or to ignore them.

2. *Using barriers at the time of fertility.* The use of a condom, diaphram, foams, jelly or spermicidal suppository in association with the Ovulation Method is contraindicated. First of all, the use of these additional methods will cause difficulty in making good mucus observations. Most condoms are prelubricated causing obvious difficulties and, of course, the foam, jellys and suppositories cause discharges. The use of barrier methods at the time of fertility also lowers the effectiveness of the Ovulation Method as a means of avoiding pregnancy. With fertility-focused use of a barrier method, a higher pregnancy rate can be anticipated. We have observed a number of pregnancies occurring under these circumstances in couples who did not take this advice. The use of a barrier method at the time of fertility is also a form of genital contact. Since the pregnancy rate is higher, we would view this as a form of achieving related behavior. The use of condoms or other forms of barrier methods also significantly reduce the pleasure and satisfaction which occurs with intercourse.

3. *A lack of spousal support in the use of the method.* It is not unusual for the use of the Ovulation Method to be initiated primarily by the woman. If that has occurred, her spouse may not be as supportive of the method as she is enthused about it. It is also true, however, that the male may be the prime mover toward the use of the method and the woman is less supportive.

If one or the other spouse is not supportive, the couple should verbalize their feelings. This lack of support, as with so many things, can only be dealt with if it is properly understood. This also allows for sharing of feelings. The spouse who is enthusiastic about the method can then express his or her feelings and then resolution of this difficulty is halfway complete. You can also explore areas where you agree and find reasons why agreement exists. This can be a positive way of working toward resolution of the different approaches.

4. *The lack of spousal agreement in using the method.* It is not unusual for a couple to lack agreement in how they are going to use the method. One spouse may wish to use the method to achieve a pregnancy while the other one is insistent on using it to avoid a pregnancy. This clearly needs to be identified and addressed since the couple, to be successful in the use of the method, must agree on how it is to be used. You may find out that the disagreement may involve a variety of different aspects of use: pregnancy

44

intention, motivation, the use of barrier methods or other methods, etc. Identifying the source of disagreement or the issue being disagreed upon is important in moving to the resolution stage. The couple should engage in *good, open and honest communication* with regard to the issue they disagree upon. You should be challenged to move toward a resolution of your disagreement. Your teacher can be of assistance in providing you education which might assist in this resolution process.

5. *The woman who lacks confidence in her husband's ability to avoid genital contact at the time of fertility.* This is not an unusual reaction although it can be quite detrimental to the couple's growth and their use of natural family planning. This reaction is more commonly observed in older women than it is in younger women. This may be related to different attitudes which were brought into marriage several years ago that are not so often involved in early marriage today.

The woman may play an important supportive role in her husband's growth beyond what is simply a genital expression. Both spouses should be fully aware that natural family planning is *particularly liberating to men.* It allows them to go beyond societal stereotypes for male behavior which are primarily genitocentric in their orientation. If she simply accepts her point of view this could actually be counterproductive to their growth.

6. *Oral-genital contact or masurbation as an "alternative" form of genital expression during the time of fertility.* First of all, it should be stressed that oral-genital contact or masturbation are not what is meant by the development of "new patterns of sexual interaction." The couple should again explore their feelings with regard to this form of genital behavior. This form of behavior is *self* motivated and puts the genital relationship out of balance, it stimulates "one partner domination". In addition, these forms of behavior are inherently frustrating and are unsatisfying. You should be encouraged to abandon this form of behavior and rely more upon the full expression of your genital sexual lives. Only by comparing a truly satisfying form of genital expression can you realize that what you were experiencing previously was actually unsatisfying.

CHAPTER 8

LONG TERM FOLLOW UP

The Ovulation Method should be viewed as a *permanent method* of family planning. Since it can be used throughout a woman's reproductive life, it can be used from the beginning of marriage through the many years when achieving and avoiding pregnancy will be necessary. As you embark on its use, you should realize that there will be times when it will be necessary to make contact with your natural family planning teacher or center for additional instruction. Your natural family planning teacher or center is properly trained for providing you the type of instruction, guidance and support which you will need during this period of time. It is ultimately the responsibility of the couple to maintain this contact. However, we want you to know that the natural family planning programs are structured in such a way so that your needs can be met.

To assist you in this, this chapter outlines several of the reasons it may be necessary for you to contact your natural family planning teacher or center, reasons why it is important to continue charting during the whole of your reproductive life and reasons it is important to come for follow up.

REASONS TO CONTACT NFP TEACHER OR CENTER

Couples who use natural family planning should be aware of those situations where they should make certain to contact their natural family planning teacher or center. Such situations would inlcude:

1. When it is necessary to make an appointment or obtain a new chart or book of stamps.
2. Whenever you have any questions related to the method or when you need updating.
3. If you become pregnant. With *each pregnancy* the client should undergo a *pregnancy evaluation*. A pregnancy evaluation will help establish the circumstances of the pregnancy and the dating of the pregnancy which will be important for you to have for your doctor.
4. Any change in Intention: Use which your teacher may be of assistance to you in clarifying.
5. Any questions you might have relative to the general field of reproductive health.
6. If you are looking for a referral for medical or spiritual counselling, or support, the natural family planning center is an excellent place to call.
7. If a speaker is needed.

Pregnancy evaluation can be, in many instances, the *very best* means of dating the pregnancy. From an obstetrical point of view, this is very helpful. At the same time, through a pregnancy evaluation, the couple will have their successful use of the method reinforced or, if the pregnancy occurred without adequate explanation, it can be helpful in clarifying those circumstances. In addition, the pregnancy evaluation can establish the support of the natural family planning teacher and center for the couple during the course of their pregnancy.

Ultimately, the long term use of natural family planning will require that support and encouragement be provided couples from all aspects of their life. As the future of natural family planning evolves, programs of this nature will be developed and will be critical to its eventual success.

REASONS FOR CONTINUED CHARTING

One of the first questions many people ask is "Do we have to continue charting for the rest of our lives?" The very simple answer to that question is yes. Reasons why continued charting is so important to the successful use of the method can be outlined as follows:

1. It is vital to the ultimate successful use of the method.
2. The chart is an excellent health record. It allows for the proper dating of pregnancies and also for the identification of some forms of gynecologic disease.
3. Continued charting will add confidence to the use of the method for both of the spouses.
4. The availability of the chart aids the couple in *mutually* carrying out their decision making.
5. The availability of the chart allows the husband an opportunity for participating more fully in the decision making process.
6. Charting should be considered an easy task. Thus, from a realistic point of view, it is a relatively minor contribution for the ongoing successful use of the method.

REASONS TO COME FOR FOLLOW UP

All couples who use the method should know that ongoing follow-up is important to the overall successful use of natural family planning. The reasons for this are:

1. It is helpful to have a periodic review of the charting, observations and instructions so that you do not become complacent in your use of the method.
2. The natural family planning teacher is an important source of support and encouragement which is necessary to your ongoing utilization of natural family planning.
3. The ongoing, long term follow-up is an excellent form of updating. Only in this way can the latest information on developments in natural family planning be provided to you.
4. As a normal course of events, you will develop questions as you continue to use the method and this allows for the questions to be answered.
5. As you change reproductive categories, throughout the course of your reproductive life, such changes really mandate continued teacher input.

CHAPTER 9

EFFECTIVENESS OF THE OVULATION METHOD
(CREIGHTON MODEL)

The Ovulation Method (Creighton Model) is a *highly reliable* method of family planning. Because this method is not a method of contraception and can be used to either achieve *or* avoid pregnancy, the statistical measure of its effectiveness must take that fact into account. The new user of the Ovulation Method must become used to looking at at least three basic statistical measures. The effectiveness of the method to achieve and avoid pregnancy in couples of normal fertility and the effectiveness of the method to achieve pregnancy in couples with infertility.

There have been three major effectiveness studies of the Creighton Model over the last several years. In these studies, the *method effectiveness* (as a means to avoid pregnancy) has ranged from 99.1 to 99.9 percent (see Table 9-1). If one takes into account teaching, using and/or human error, the *use effectiveness* (as a means to avoid pregnancy) ranged from 94.8 to 97.4 percent. Both of these effectiveness ratings are equal to or better than birth control pills or other drugs and devices.

As couples use the Ovulation Method, many will elect to use it to achieve pregnancy. Out of every 100 couples who enter a program to use the method to avoid pregnancy, a number of them will adopt the method as a method to achieve pregnancy and be successful in so doing during the first twelve months of use. This figure is far more flexible than the method and use effectiveness to avoid pregnancy and is reflected in the studies of the method. Thus, *the use effectiveness to achieve pregnancy* ranged from 13.1 to 28.0 percent (see Table 9-2). As a rule of thumb, one can expect that one out of five couples will use the method as a means of achieving a pregnancy during the first year of use and that four out of five pregnancies that occur in users of the method are the result of *its successful use.*

The *method effectiveness to achieve pregnancy* is higher than this. But, it is measured differently as well. This type of effectiveness is measured by evaluating couples of normal fertility as they use the time of fertility *in a given menstrual cycle.* A study recently published shows that it is *very likely* that pregnancies will be achieved within the *very first cycle* in which the time of fertility is used. Indeed, 76.0 percent of couples achieved pregnancy during the first cycle in which the time of fertility was used. It is because of this experience that we say there is no such thing as "taking a chance" when using the method.

For couples with infertility, the overall pregnancy rate runs approximately 20 to 40 percent during the first six months in which the time of fertility is consistently used. This figure will vary depending upon the type of pattern exhibited. Again, it should be pointed out, however, that with adequate medical assessment and treatment, this figure can be increased significantly.

The above data comes from three studies performed at Creighton University in Omaha, Nebraska and St. John's Mercy Medical Center, St. Louis, Missouri, St. Francis Hospital in Wichita, Kansas and St. Joseph Hospital in Houston, Texas. The three studies cumulatively involved 1,632 couples in their use of the method over 14,668 couple months of use or 1,222 couple years of use.

TABLE 9-1

METHOD AND USE-EFFECTIVENESS TO AVOID PREGNANCY
OF THE CREIGHTON MODEL NATURAL FAMILY PLANNING SYSTEM
BY ORDINAL MONTH AND CENTER CONDUCTING STUDY

ORDINAL MONTH	METHOD EFFECTIVENESS			USE-EFFECTIVENESS		
	CREIGHTON[1]	WICHITA[2]	HOUSTON[3]	CREIGHTON	WICHITA	HOUSTON
6	99.6	99.4	100.0	95.8	97.3	98.6
12	99.6	99.1	99.9	94.8	96.2	97.4
18	99.6	N/A	99.9	94.6	N/A	97.1
Year of study	1980	1985	1989	—	—	—
Number of couples	559	376	697	—	—	—
Number of couples months	4,957	2,463	7,238	—	—	—

1. Hilgers, T.W., Prebil, A.M. and Daly, K.D.: The Effectiveness of the Ovulation Method as a Means of Achieving and Avoiding Pregnancy. Presented at Education Phase III Continuing Education Conference for Natural Family Planning Practitioners, July 24, 1980, Mercy Fontenelle Center, Omaha, Nebraska.

2. Doud, J.: Use-effectiveness of the Creighton Model of NFP. Int. Rev. Nat. Fam. Plan. 9:54, 1985.

3. Howard, M.P.: Use-effectiveness of the Ovulation Method (Creighton Model) of Natural Famly Planning. St. Joseph Hospital, Houston, Texas, 1989.

TABLE 9-2

USE-EFFECTIVENESS TO ACHIEVE PREGNANCY
OF THE CREIGHTON MODEL NATURAL FAMILY PLANNING SYSTEMS
BY ORDINAL MONTH AND CENTER CONDUCTING STUDY

ORDINAL MONTH	USE-EFFECTIVENESS TO ACHIEVE		
	CREIGHTON[1]	WICHITA[2]	HOUSTON[3]
6	12.0	19.9	7.3
12	21.3	28.0	13.1
18	26.8	N/A	24.9
Year of Study	1980	1985	1989
Number of Couples	559	376	697
Number of Couple-months	4,957	2,463	7,238

1. Hilgers, T.W., Prebil, A.M. and Daly, K.D.: The Effectiveness of the Ovulation Method as a Means of Achieving and Avoiding Pregnancy. Presented at Education Phase III Continuing Education Conference for Natural Family Planning Practitioners, July 24, 1980, Mercy Fontenelle Center, Omaha, Nebraska.

2. Doud, J.: Use-effectiveness of the Creighton Model of NFP. Int. Rev. Nat. Fam. Plan. 9:54, 1985.

3. Howard, M.P.: Use-effectiveness of the Ovulation Method (Creighton Model) of Natural Famly Planning. St. Joseph Hospital, Houston, Texas, 1989.

CHAPTER 10

AN INTRODUCTION TO NAPROTECHNOLOGY

NaProTechnology is a newly emerging gynecologic and reproductive science. It can be defined as a science which devotes its medical, surgical and allied health energies and attention to *cooperating* with the natural procreative mechanisms and functions. When these mechanisms are working properly, NaProTechnology works cooperatively with them. When these mechanisms are functioning abnormally, NaProTechnology cooperates with the procreative mechanisms in producing a form of treatment which *corrects the condition, maintains the human ecology and sustains the procreative potential.*

This new science has been developed through the research efforts of the Pope Paul VI Institute for the Study of Human Reproduction in Omaha, Nebraska. It involves the orderly and systematic evaluation of the events that occur during the course of the menstrual and ovulation cycles and it has been built upon the new, standardized, *gynecologic charting record* which has become known as the *Creighton Model Natural Family Planning System* or *CrM NFP.* This charting depends upon recording the patterns of bleeding, mucus discharge and dry days. These serve as *very sensitive biomarkers for assessing the normal and abnormal of gynecologic and reproductive function.*

As with any new science, it has its own specialized terminology or vocabulary. As one studies the practical art of CrM NFP one will be able to discuss with a clear understanding the pre-Peak phase and the post-Peak phase of the cycle, the length of the mucus cycle, the classification of the mucus cycle, the intensity of the menstrual flow, the differing types of discharges, and all of the various patterns which an understanding of NaProTechnology elicits.

As one understands this new science better, one will be able to identify cervical *eversions* and *erosions* (inflammatory reactions of the cervix), differing types of *ovarian cysts,* causes of *unusual bleeding* and associated causes of various reproductive disorders including *infertility, miscarriage* and *ectopic pregnancy.* One will be able to *date* the beginning of the pregnancy from the *true beginning* (the time of conception) instead of the usual *false beginning* which is used currently (the first day of the last menstrual period). One will understand how to *cooperatively evaluate* the endocrinology (hormone status) of the menstrual cycle and provide true *progesterone replacement therapy.* This allows for a more accurate and precise evaluation of ovarian function and the subsequent treatment of abnormal ovarian function. One will better understand *the effects of stress* on the menstrual cycle. One will learn how to effectively treat *premenstrual syndrome (PMS)* and understand some of the indications and reasons for the use of progesterone support in pregnancy.

It is essential that women keep good gynecologic charting records. These records are best kept through the use of the Creighton Model Natural Family Planning System. Because this system is *standardized* and *objective,* it provides very accurate information. Thus, as one uses this system as a natural method of family planning, one also is using it as a *reproductive health maintenance system.*

NaProTechnology is a science which empowers women to take control of their fertility, understand their natural sequences of fertility and infertility and *be several steps ahead* in the evaluation and eventual treatment of gynecologic and reproductive abnormalities.

While this charting system *does not prove* that certain conditions exist, it does indicate with a *reasonable degree of likelihood* that the possibility of such exists. *Further medical evaluation may be necessary once the high risk individual is identified.* Your Natural Family Planning Practitioner will be able to assist you in identifying these kinds of difficulties and arrange for referral to medical assistance. *One should expect to identify problems in their early stages* and treat them effectively before they become long term problems.

As one understands NaProTechnology and adopts it as a way of life, one will learn how *to reduce* the number of surgical procedures performed for ovarian cysts, how to reduce significantly the number of hysterectomies performed, how to *better evaluate* and subsequently *treat* infertility, miscarriage and ectopic pregnancy, and how to generally participate in your own *gynecologic health maintenance.*

Indeed, this is the *contemporary approach to women's health care.* It is *medically safe,* respectful to the *dignity* of women and *effective* in what it says it is able to do.

This chapter is designed to introduce you to the potential that NaProTechnology has for providing you with this type of information. A more detailed presentation of NaProTechnology can be found in the following book: Hilgers, TW: *The Medical Applications of Natural Family Planning.* Pope Paul VI Institute Press, Omaha, NE, 1991, ($29.95). Physicians who are trained in NaProTechnology are referred to as *Natural Family Planning Medical Consultants.*

CHRONIC DISCHARGES

Women who have an inflammatory condition of the cervix may experience a very characteristic discharge pattern. This inflammatory condition is commonly associated with cervical *eversion or ectropion,* a cervical *erosion* or a *cervicitis.* These conditions may cause a discharge to occur at specific times during the menstrual cycle. With the help of your natural family planning teacher, who is knowledgable in the specific criteria which have been developed to identify these cervical inflammations, the woman can identify the presence of such an inflammation from her natural family planning chart with at least *75 percent accuracy.*

There are a variety of different medical treatments for this condition if it is properly identified. The one that we have used most recently is a low intensity cauterization of the cervix (using an instrument called a Hyfrecator). This is less damaging to the cervix than the usual cryosurgical systems which require freezing of the cervix. There are, of course, other management plans which can be helpful such as using progesterone vaginal capsules during the post-Peak phase of the menstrual cycle. If medical assistance is not available, your teacher will assist you in the use of pre- and post-peak yellow stamps.

COOPERATIVE HORMONE EVALUATION
OF THE MENSTRUAL CYCLE

One of the difficulties in evaluating the hormonal aspects of menstrual and ovulatory function is the fact that the various hormones of the menstrual cycle are produced in differing quantities during the course of the cycle. Indeed, the hallmark of the menstrual cycle hormones is that they are not the same from day to day (see Figure 10-1).

Characteristic of the menstrual cycle is the rise in estrogen which occurs four to five days prior to the time of ovulation and peaks about 36 hours before. In addition, the estrogen level rises again during the post-ovulatory phase of the menstrual cycle along with an increase in progesterone. The progesterone hormone, however, increases *only* following ovulation.

**HORMONES
OF THE
MENSTRUAL CYCLE**

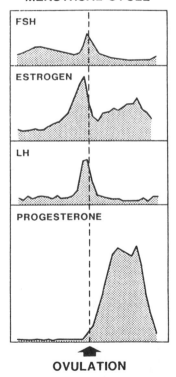

OVULATION

Figure 10-1   The hormones of the menstrual cycle

It is also true that such hormones as FSH, LH, Testosterone, Prolactin and Beta Endorphin have cyclic variations throughout the course of the cycle and thus can be more difficult to assess without an adequate understanding of the events of the cycle itself.

It is *common medical practice* to assess the hormones of the menstrual cycle by drawing the hormonal test based on the day of the cycle. For example it is not uncommon for a physician to order a progesterone level, testing for the adequacy of the post-ovulatory phase, on day 22 of the cycle. The physician presumes that most menstrual cycles are 28 days in duration. However, only five to ten percent of cycles are 28 days long and, thus, drawing the hormone levels at that time of the cycle is often not very productive. The progesterone level may be extremely low or it may be in the preovulatory range giving the false impression that there is an inadequate luteal phase or that the woman is not ovulating. The same can be said for the measurement of the other hormones of the menstrual cycle. *What perhaps is even more important is the need to look at the reproductive hormones as they are produced over a period of time.* In other words it is better to measure a *profile* of the hormone production than it is to rely on a single measurement.

This timing of the hormone assessment can be accomplished if the physician has access to a simple system of determining when the woman is both pre- and post-ovulatory. This simple system is found in the CrM NFP. With this NaProTechnique, the woman is able to identify her Peak day, a day which is closely associated with the timing of ovulation. This is one of the keys to a good understanding of NaProTechnology.

Thus, if one uses the Peak day to look at both the pre- and post-ovulatory hormones, one can then be more accurate with regard to the hormonal assessment of the menstrual cycle.

The progesterone levels at various stages of the post-Peak phase of the cycle in a group of patients of normal fertility and a group of patients with infertility are shown in Figure 10-2.

Figure 10-2

Progesterone Levels at Various Stages of the Post Peak Phase:
Normal Controls and All Infertility

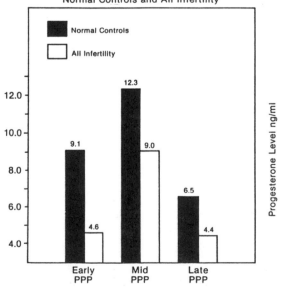

Stage of Post-Peak Phase (PPP)

This form of cooperative hormone evaluation of the menstrual cycle is a critical, *basic principle* to the proper assessment of the ovarian and pituitary events. But because these simple charting systems are not often used, irrelevant test results are obtained, false or inappropriate interpretations of test results are observed and costs are inflated.

Thus, this simple technique allows for a good understanding of the menstrual cycle to be obtained for both the physician and the patient. Such an evaluation is essential to the basic principle of gaining a good understanding of underlying hormonal events which may be abnormal.

COOPERATIVE PROGESTERONE REPLACEMENT THERAPY (CPRT)

Another key element to NaProTechnology, which is especially important from a therapeutic point of view, is the concept of *Cooperative Progesterone Replacement Therapy (CPRT)*. The concept is basically a simple one and can be outlined in the following points:

1. Progesterone is produced in a cyclic fashion *only* in the post-ovulatory phase of the cycle (see Figure 10-1).

2. True progesterone replacement therapy must, therefore, be provided *only* during the post-ovulatory phase of the cycle.

3. The pre-ovulatory phase of the cycle is *variable* in length.

4. Therefore, one must have a simple, but reliable means of determining when the patient is in the post-ovulatory phase of the cycle.

5. The Peak day is a reliable, reproducible sign of ovulation and is *the hallmark* for the woman to know that she is entering the post-ovulatory phase of her cycle.

Starting progesterone therapy on a *given day* of the cycle is inappropriate because of the variability of the pre-ovulatory phase of the cycle. But the Peak day is a reliable sign of the day of ovulation and thus, using the post-Peak phase of the cycle as an indicator for the use of progesterone provides a means by which one can identify the time when progesterone is *needed* and is *therapeutic*. Providing progesterone in this way is what we refer to as Cooperative Progesterone Replacement Therapy (CPRT).

Progesterone can be provided in this way using a variety of different systems. One can use progesterone suppositories, progesterone vaginal capsules, injections of progesterone or human chorionic gonadotropin (HCG).

THE IDENTIFICATION AND TREATMENT OF OVARIAN CYSTS

Ovarian cysts can often be identified in patients using CrM NFP. The ovarian cysts that can be identified are those that are functional or physiologic in their pathophysiology. Thus, *persistent follicular cysts* or *persistent luteal cysts* are the most common ones identified.

With regard to ovarian cysts, it is important to recognize that there are other causes of ovarian cysts than simply the functional variety. Thus, it is important, when dealing with ovarian cysts to *not presume that they are totally benign. Careful follow-up and ongoing assessment is critical.*

Having said that, however, the overwhelming majority of ovarian cysts seen in a reproductive age group are going to be benign functional cysts. By understanding the basic principles of NaProTechnology, one has some additional information with which to evaluate the ovarian cyst. *In many cases, this results in a reduced need for surgical intervention.* As a general rule, *women with functional cysts do not need surgery.* There are some exceptions to this, but those exceptions are related to either internal hemorrhage, significant internal bleeding or incapacitating pain (both of which are quite rare).

The tragedy, quite frankly, is that a number of women, especially young women are operated on for ovarian cysts when such operations are unnecessary.

With a follicular ovarian cyst, the CrM NFP chart will reveal a prolonged Peak-type mucus discharge and a delayed Peak day. In addition, this is often associated with chronic pelvic pain which is usually on one side but it may be on both sides.

A persistent luteal cyst (Luteinized Unruptured Follicle Syndrome—LUF Syndrome) is one in which the follicle grows and develops to the time of ovulation but ovulation, the rupture of the follicle, does not occur. Thus, the follicle remains unruptured and a cyst continues to form and usually increases in size during the remainder of the cycle. If the woman is charting her cycles using CrM NFP, the post-Peak phase of the cycle may be prolonged 16 or more days in duration. If this occurs, it is suspicious for the presence of the LUF. In the absence of pregnancy and in the absence of the misidentification of the Peak day, the interpretation of this chart as one which reflects a persistent luteal cyst will be accurate in the overwhelming majority of cases. However, good ultrasound evaluation can be very useful in further evaluating this.

It is common for physicians to treat both of these types of cysts with birth control pills. However, this is a suppressive form of treatment and is contrary to the best principles of NaProTechnology. In addition, it is unnecessary given an understanding of the CrM NFP Systems.

The usual treatment of these cysts is to give an injection of progesterone which causes the pain to disappear and the cyst to disappear as well.

THE EFFECTS OF STRESS

Stress has an enormous impact on the ovulation and menstrual cycles. The stress may be physical or emotional and it may be *acute* or *chronic*.

A variety of different patterns can be observed in women who are under stress. First of all, one can have the delayed appearance of the mucus cycle and a delay in the observation of the Peak day when an acute stress occurs right around the time when one would expect to be ovulating. In effect, the ovulation is suppressed and delayed and thus the mucus cycle is delayed along with it.

In other cases, the mucus cycle may be very prolonged lasting upwards to three or four weeks in duration with the Peak day also delayed. This may also be observed with acute stress occurring during the middle of the mucus buildup.

Some women will observe limited mucus cycles or dry cycles as the result of chronic stress. This is quite common in the women who experience infertility, miscarriage, tubal pregnancy or other reproductive disorders.

PREMENSTRUAL SYNDROME (PMS)

Premenstrual Syndrome (PMS) is a condition where a series of symptoms occur on a regular and routine basis during the premenstrual phase of the menstrual cycle. In its more advanced stages, *it can be a very debilitating condition* for those women who suffer from it.

PMS is generally considered to be a *progesterone deficiency condition*. However, studies showing progesterone defiency have been conflicting. Other studies have shown decreased levels of Beta-endorphins during the post-ovulatory or premenstrual phase of the menstrual cycle suggesting that this may play a role in its cause.

Treatment for the condition has revolved around various plans of nutritional support, stress management and the post-ovulatory support of the luteal phase with progesterone. However, the success of these approaches to treatment have varied and its treatment remains controversial.

The tragedy of this condition is that the majority of physicians either deny that it exists or simply believe that women periodically have emotional swings that are normal. On a number of occasions I have heard physicians say, "If a woman presents with these symptoms, just give her some Valium since all women have this problem eventually."

Equally disturbing is the feminist notion that recognizing PMS as a real condition is in someway denigrating to women. In fact, it could be strongly argued that the denial of PMS is denigrating to women and recognizing that it exists and working towards its successful treatment is what can best help women with these symptoms. In fact, as we will show, women can be virtually cured of these symptoms with the use of Cooperative Progesterone Replacement Therapy (CPRT) and NaProTechnology.

PMS is a grouping of symptoms which, for the most part, begin seven to ten days prior to the onset of menstruation. However, these symptoms can sometimes also be present around the time of ovulation and again during the early days of the menstrual cycle. *Some mild symptoms one or two days prior to menstruation should not be considered PMS.* These symptoms usually include bloating, fatigue, irritability, depression, teariness, breast tenderness, carbohydrate craving, weight gain, headache and/or insomnia.

The premenstrual appearance of migraine headaches can be impressive and its subsequent treatment can be extraordinary. Anxiety, confusional states, dizziness, clumsiness, even suicidal tendencies can be observed. On a number of occasions, the author has observed the mistaken diagnosis of depressive psychosis or manic-depressive psychosis made by well thought of psychiatrists in women whose primary problem was PMS.

Fundamentally, the treatment for this condition is to provide progesterone support during the premenstrual phase of the cycle. This is done by providing Cooperative Progesterone Replacement Therapy (CPRT). A thorough hormone evaluation of the post-ovulatory phase of the cycle is essential, however, prior to beginning treatment.

EVALUATING INFERTILITY, MISCARRIAGE AND ECTOPIC PREGNANCY

Infertility is a serious problem thought by many to be on the increase at the present time. All too often, physicians do not take the condition seriously and treat the patients as if it is "all in their head." And yet the inability to freely use one's procreative capabilities in the generation of new life causes a considerable amount of heartbreak (both physical, emotional and spiritual) in those couples who are confronted with it.

NaProTechnology has a great deal to offer those couples who have a reproductive disorder. It assists them in identifying the peak time of their fertility. The Ovulation Method is *the most precise method* currently available for identifying the peak time of fertility and is *far superior* to the urinary test kits. In this way it assists in *the treatment* of the infertility problem. In addition, NaProTechnology can be very helpful in the overall evaluation of the reproductive disorder itself.

The evaluation of a reproductive disorder is enhanced with the use of CrM NFP charting. The standardized mucus observations and the excellent records of bleeding episodes and dry days become an excellent ingredient in the evaluation and eventual treatment of the couple afflicted with the disorder.

Such things as *limited mucus cycles, dry cycles, short post-Peak phases, premenstrual spotting, post-menstrual brown bleeding* and *light periods* are all more common in women who have a reproductive disorder. Thus, by keeping these charts, *one plays an active role in the actual evaluation of the disorder.*

Based on current evidence, all of these changes are apparently due to aberrations in the hormonal sequence of events that control ovulation. Besides the abnormalities in progesterone and estrogen production and most likely FSH and LH, there is the likelihood that a number of receptors are abnormally functioning as well. This would be particularly true for the estrogen and progesterone receptors.

If the mucus cycle is *limited* in duration and amount it suggests an increased risk situation for *infertility, miscarriage and ectopic pregnancy.* In fact, by observing a limited mucus cycle, one can identify the high risk situation and, with proper medical management, reduce the chances of such occurring.

If *premenstrual spotting* exists (three or more days of light, very light or brown bleeding prior to menstruation), this is highly suggestive of low progesterone levels during that post-ovulatory phase of the cycle.

Tail end brown bleeding at the end of menses also is the result of an irregular sloughing of the lining of the uterus and is due to low progesterone levels during the previous cycle.

If the post-Peak phase is too short in duration, seven days or less in duration, this suggests that the post-ovulatory phase is not adequate to sustain a pregnancy.

If the post-Peak phase is prolonged (16 days or longer in duration) it suggests that the woman is experiencing the Unruptured Follicle Syndrome which means that the cycle is anovulatory.

As one begins to understand the different dimensions of the *abnormal mucus cycles,* the *premenstrual spotting,* the *prolonged or short post-Peak phases,* etc., one can better understand how this relates to the infertility problem. The charting usually suggests a hormonal abnormality or a problem with ovulation. However, underlying these conditions are often other conditions such as *endometriosis* or *pelvic adhesive disease.*

The treatment of various reproductive disorders depends upon being able to *cooperatively treat* the ovulation cycles. NaProTechnology recognizes the fact that the human body is more efficient in being able to orchestrate ovulation and support for pregnancy than we are able to, as physicians, artificially construct. While recognizing that abnormalities may exist, the treatment programs are designed to cooperate with the already existing function with an attempt to enhance or improve that function at the appropriate time during the cycle. The CrM NFP standardized charting is the key to being able to accomplish this.

UNUSUAL BLEEDING

Unusual bleeding is defined as that bleeding which is interpreted *by the woman* as being any bleeding *other* than a normal (usual) menstrual flow. *A true menstrual flow* follows an *ovulatory event,* and it is very characteristic.

An ovulatory event is defined as any event which actually is ovulation or *mimics* ovulation. Thus, any situation in which a corpus luteum is formed and luteal phase progesterone is produced will be followed by a very characteristic sloughing of the lining of the uterus which is called menstruation. The menstrual event is a very characteristic experience and can be defined by women as being either "usual" or "unusual".

The characteristics of a menstrual bleeding episode exist in its pattern to begin as a lighter bleeding and then build to more heavy bleeding and then taper again. We call this *crescendo-decrescendo bleeding.*

The natural family planning teacher will be able to assist the natural family planning client couple with the interpretation of their bleeding episodes and get them to proper medical assistance.

DATING THE BEGINNING OF PREGNANCY

Even with all of the available technology, one of the puzzles of modern obstetrics is that the doctor has not yet learned how to date the beginning of a pregnancy. The traditional way of measuring the beginning of pregnancy is to measure it from the first day of the last menstrual period. On average, this will be approximately two weeks prior to the actual date of the pregnancy itself.

Pregnancy can be measured in two ways. The most common is measuring the gestational age of the pregnancy. The gestational age of the pregnancy is measured from the first day of the last menstrual period. In this way of dating the pregnancy, the pregnancy is 40 weeks in duration (on average) instead of the *actual 38 weeks.* In other words, it dates the pregnancy, on average two weeks longer than it actually is.

The other way of measuring the dates of the pregnancy is to measure the *fetal age.* The fetal age of the pregnancy is measured from the time of conception or the estimated time of conception. When measuring the pregnancy in this fashion, the pregnancy is 38 weeks in gestation or two weeks shorter than gestational age dates. The fetal age, of course, is *the actual age* or date of the pregnancy.

Historically, the doctor focused on the first day of the last menstrual period for two reasons. First of all, the menstrual flow was a fairly dramatic symptom which the woman could be expected to remember. In addition, it was easy to teach her to record the first day of the last menstrual period so that when that information was elicited by the physician, at a later time, it would be available.

However, in the midst of all this, the doctor and many women missed the point that the cervical mucus discharge is very much *a flow* in the same fashion as the menstrual flow. When one is charting the Ovulation Method, one can date the pregnancy accurately from the actual or estimated time of conception. Therefore, one can date the pregnancy according to *its true date* or in fetal age terms. This is measured by evaluating the acts of intercourse that occur *during the time of fertility* and establishing an estimated time of conception. Again, your natural family planning teacher has expertise in being able to assist you with that.

It is true that a *cervical mucus* discharge is not a "high tech" idea. However, it is an *incredibly good biomarker.* Everyone concerned needs to recognize the accuracy of this bioassay system and *the ease* with which such information is obtained so that it's benefits can better be incorporated into obstetrical practice.

PROGESTERONE SUPPORT IN PREGNANCY

As one better understands those events which lead upto the beginning of pregnancy, one can recognize that events occurring around the time of ovulation and in the early days following ovulation have an impact on the subsequent growth and development of the pregnancy. The use of progesterone in pregnancy must be recognized as being important in those pregnancies where the progesterone production is low during the immediate post-ovulation phase of the menstrual cycle.

We have studied, for several years, the production of progesterone during the course of pregnancy. We have found that progesterone support in pregnancy can be helpful in those patients with previous *infertility, miscarriage* or *ectopic pregnancy*. In addition, individuals who can be considered candidates for progesterone evaluation and subsequent supplementation are those who have had a *previous abruptio placentae, previous stillbirth, pregnancy induced hypertension, previous prematurity, previous premature rupture of the membranes, previous or current intrauterine growth retardation, hyperirritability of the uterus, congenital uterine anomaly* or patients with *cervical cerclage*.

Supportive measures in pregnancy, which are safe and effective, are a natural component of a good understanding of NaProTechnology. With progesterone support, only the natural progesterone should be used. While progesterone support is not a "miracle cure" for the previously listed problems, it can be a component to help subsequent pregnancies. Additional research on this subject is currently being done and the results will be forthcoming.

THE FUTURE

Our continued study of NaProTechnology holds a bright and beckoning future. How much progress we make will depend to a great extent on the depth of our willingness and the breadth of our vision.

Currently, we are able to identify women who have continuous discharges earlier than in the past. Because of this, we can identify abnormalities of the cervix and endometrium and, with unusual bleeding patterns, we will eventually see women with endometrial cancers in their very earliest stages. As we learn more and more how to recognize and treat the various causes of unusual bleeding, we will be able to make a real dent in the number of hysterectomies performed. It is even theoretically possible to identify some women who might be at high risk for *breast cancer*. More research is needed in this area.

As we learn how to recognize and treat the various ovarian cysts, especially the functional ones, we will make a significant impact on the numbers of inappropriate surgical procedures performed; surgical procedures which leave their own mark of pelvic adhesions and scarring and its potentially devastating effect on future fertility.

With our ability to identify when a pregnancy begins by accurately estimating the time of conception rather than relying upon the older techniques of counting from the first day of the last menstrual period, we should be able to decrease some forms of obstetrical interference.

As we look at women who suffer from PMS and all the controversy that exists with regard to its existence and treatment, we should be able to eventually lay that issue to rest. And with that, we should be able to provide a reproducible and effective therapeutic program for women suffering from this problem.

As we recognize more and more what CrM NFP can do for patients with reproductive disorders, we should be able to provide different types of advice than what is currently provided. For example, we should be able to recognize people who are high risk for infertility, miscarriage or ectopic pregnancy before they even experience those problems. If we can do this, then our advice to those patients would change. They would be able to begin testing their fertility long before, perhaps, they had planned. Clearly, if there is a problem, the earlier one identifies it and treats it the more successful one will be.

The only requirement to make this equation functional is *good education* in the practical applications of *gynecologic health maintenance*. Women need to see that the simple observations and charting of the CrM NFP System are essential for good and healthy family planning purposes *as well as* good *gynecologic record keeping*. They need to recognize that CrM NFP and NaProTechnology *empowers* them to be in control of their reproductive health. *Your CrM NFP teacher will help you towards that end.*

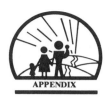

APPENDIX

SPECIAL CIRCUMSTANCES

The instructions of the Ovulation Method vary from one circumstance to another. Generally, these variations are used only temporarily until the basic method instructions are implemented. The instructions for these various situations are referred to as *special method instructions.* In this appendix, many of these various circumstances are discussed and their special instructions outlined. This should be thought of as your "home reference" to these instructions. *However, keep in mind that when you enter one of these circumstances, you should see your Natural Family Planning Practitioner or Instructor for further guidance.*

While most users will be particularly interested in the special circumstances they currently find themselves in, there are several items in this chapter which *every Ovulation Method user should be thoroughly familiar with.* These include the *note on the pre-Peak instructions,* the *seminal fluid instruction,* the *arousal fluid instruction, early ovulation, "double" Peak* and *"split" Peak.*

COMING OFF BIRTH CONTROL PILLS

The following special considerations should be applied to those couples who are coming off birth control pills.

1. Stop the pill immediately after the introductory session. Withdrawal bleeding should be anticipated within a few days after stopping the pill.

2. The interval between the time of the withdrawal bleeding and the first normal menses may be longer than the woman's usual cycle interval. In addition, the first normal period will usually be heavier than pill "periods".

3. The first ovulation following cessation of the pill may be more painful than usual.

4. The woman may be temporarily (or even permanently) anovulatory after stopping the pill resulting in a long period of time in which ovulation and menses does not occur. Such an occurrence poses little difficulty in using the Ovulation Method as a method to avoid pregnancy. The instructions relative to anovulatory states such as breastfeeding should be followed in this circumstance. However, persistent post-Pill anovulation can be a cause of infertility and if it persists longer than six months after cessation of the pill, the woman should see her physician.

5. Once the woman begins in cycles, the pre-Peak phase of the cycle may be more variable in length than usual.

6. The post-Peak phase of the cycle may also be more variable in length during the initial serveral months of charting.

7. If there is a delay in the return of ovulation, the woman may experience a variable return of Peak-type mucus typical of anovulatory conditions.

8. Since avoiding genital contact may be initially difficult after stopping birth control pills, it is necessary for the couple to work on the creation of other non-genital expressions of their love (see chapter 7).

SPECIAL INSTRUCTIONS

A. If it is the intention to avoid pregnancy, intercourse should always be at the end of the infertile days through the first normal menstrual cycle.

B. The basic pre-Peak method instructions apply through the first normal menstrual cycle.

C. After the first normal menstrual cycle, the basic pre- and post-Peak method instructions apply.

D. If anovulation occurs or a continuous discharge is present, manage as for those two conditions.

Some charting examples of what might be observed in women coming off of birth control pills can be found by reviewing Figures A-1, A-2, A-3, A-9 and A-10.

A NOTE ABOUT "NORMAL CYCLES"

A normal cycle is one in which the woman has confidently identified the Peak day and a usual menstrual flow has occurred 8 to 16 days later.

A NOTE ON THE PRE-PEAK INSTRUCTIONS

When the use of the *pre-Peak instructions* is referred to, it means that intercourse is limited to the *end* of the infertile days and that the instructions related to both Peak type and non-Peak type mucus are recommended. If the couple has not passed *the* Peak day, the couple is still pre-Peak and intercourse should occur, if the couple intends to avoid pregnancy, on infertile dry days only and then only at the end of the day. Any mucus which is observed is considered fertile and the instructions are followed as they would apply to that type of discharge.

BREASTFEEDING

Suckling an infant at the breast produces a physiological suppression of ovulation which may continue for an extended period of time. However, fertility can return prior to the return of menstruation.

Important in understanding the instructions as they apply to breastfeeding is an understanding of the differences between total and partial breastfeeding.

Total Breastfeeding - All of the infants nutritional sustenance (except for occasional sips of water) is received from the breast.

Partial Breastfeeding - When supplemental feeding is begun, as an addition to breastfeeding, the woman is defined to be partially breastfeeding.

The best time for the breastfeeding couple to be introduced to the Ovulation Method is during the last three months of pregnancy. At that time, they should attend an introductory session. In this way, they will be prepared for the post-partum period and they can proceed directly to a schedule of follow-up appointments (see Figure A-3).

If totally breastfeeding
1. You should begin charting when the bleeding decreases (usually three weeks post-partum).

2. The first follow-up should be scheduled at 5 weeks post-partum, at which time, you will have two weeks of charting to discuss.

A. You should consider the first eight weeks (the first 56 days after the birthdate of the baby) as infertile.

B. If you do not come into the program until after the eighth week postpartum, then, genital contact must be avoided for two weeks (if completely dry during this time) or four weeks (if mucus is apparent).

C. Intercourse should always occur at the end of the day through the first normal menstrual cycle.

D. The basic pre-Peak instructions are applicable during this period of time.

IF PARTIALLY BREASTFEEDING
A. The first eight weeks after the birthdate of the baby are not considered infertile.

B. You should avoid genital contact for one month to learn the mucus symptom with confidence.

C. If you are avoiding pregnancy, intercourse should occur always at the end of the day through the first normal menstrual cycle.

D. The basic pre-Peak instructions apply.

Once Menses Returns
1. When menses returns, you should make an appointment to see your Natural Family Planning teacher.

When weaning commences, a variable return of Peak-type mucus may be experienced. This is due to the rising and falling levels of estrogen which occur during this period of time with the return of ovulatory function. As the estrogen levels rise, Peak-type mucus is produced. As they fall, this type of mucus disappears. The instructions of the Ovulation Method allow you to navigate this period usually without great difficulty.

POSTPARTUM - NOT BREASTFEEDING
The earliest ovulation reported in the medical literature following childbirth in the absence of breastfeeding has been at 27 days. Therefore, no automatic time of infertility can be presupposed in this group of women.

The best time to be introduced to the Ovulation Method is during the last three months of pregnancy. The following instructions should be used for this reproductive category (see Figure A-4).

1. Charting should begin when the bleeding decreases, usually three to four weeks following delivery.

2. The couple should avoid genital contact for the first four weeks of charting so the woman can develop confidence in her observations.

3. The first follow-up should be scheduled for two weeks after charting has begun.

SPECIAL INSTRUCTIONS

A. If it is the intention to avoid pregnancy, intercourse should always be at the end of the infertile days through the first normal menstrual cycle.

B. The basic pre-Peak method instructions apply through the first normal menstrual cycle.

C. After the first normal menstrual cycle, the basic pre- and post-Peak method instructions apply.

POST-ABORTION (MISCARRIAGE)

Women who have had a spontaneous abortion (miscarriage), induced abortion or ectopic pregnancy, will have very little suppression of ovulation after the loss. Ovulation can return within two weeks. Therefore, the following instructions apply to this reproductive category:

1. Charting should begin when the bleeding decreases. This is usually within one week following the incident.

2. The couple should avoid genital contact for the first four weeks of charting so the woman can develop confidence in her observations.

3. The first follow-up should be scheduled for two weeks after charting has begun.

SPECIAL INSTRUCTIONS

A. If it is the intention to avoid pregnancy, intercourse should always be at the end of the infertile days through the first normal menstrual cycle.

B. The basic pre-Peak method instructions apply through the first normal menstrual cycle.

C. After the first normal menstrual cycle, the basic pre- and post-Peak method instructions apply.

Whenever a woman suffers a miscarriage, induced abortion or ectopic pregnancy, there is a sense of loss which follows. For each of the situations, there is a grieving process which the woman, her husband and even members of the family will go through. Your natual family planning teacher is aware of that process and support will be provided to the couple during this period of time.

PREMENOPAUSE

The menopause is defined as the cessation of menstrual flow. The time leading up to the menopause is called the pre-menopause.

The Ovulation Method is a great advance for couples in this age group. It gives them the necessary security which they desire in their family planning. Although the menstrual cycles tend to become shorter and more irregular the instructions will carry them through without much difficulty.

The following are important instructions for this reproductive category (see Figure A-5).

1. The cycle patterns may be irregular and/or anovulatory.

2. The mucus patterns may be more irregular with more mucus "patches" and a variable return of Peak-type mucus observed.

3. The pre-Peak phase of the cycle may be shorter than usual. Therefore, it is necessary to watch for early ovulation by being certain to observe for the presence or absence of mucus during menses.

4. The post-Peak phase may be irregular in length from cycle to cycle.

5. Unusual bleeding may be more frequently observed so the instructions regarding unusual bleeding may be more applicable.

6. The menopause can be said to have been reached when one year passes without a period.

INSTRUCTIONS
A. Basic method instructions apply

IMPORTANT

At any time that a woman in this age group develops unusual bleeding, a continuous discharge, intermenstrual bleeding or a discharge that is malodorous, she should see her doctor.

INFERTILITY

Natural family planning offers hope to the couple with an infertility problem because it assists them in identifying the Peak time of their fertility. This is particularly true for the Ovulation Method. The Ovulation Method is the most precise method currently available for identifying the Peak time of fertility. In this way it assists in the treatment of the infertility problem. In addition, the Ovulation Method can be very helpful in the overall evaluation of the infertility problem itself.

A number of patterns can now be described as a preliminary look at the use of the Ovulation Method in the evaluation of infertility. These patterns include dry cycles, limited mucus cycles and normal mucus cycles (see Figure A-6).

A. Dry cycles - A dry cycle is one in which there is no cervical mucus discharge observed throughout the course of the menstrual cycle.

B. Limited mucus cycles - In limited mucus cycles, the amount of cervical mucus discharge is significantly reduced. Both dry and limited mucus cycles are generally associated with inadequate ovarian function.

C. Normal mucus cycles - In normal mucus cycles, the amount of cervical mucus discharge is normal.

The following are important considerations for this reproductive category:

1. The infertility couple should avoid all genital contact during the first *complete* menstrual cycle. It is as important to the infertility couple as it is to the couple who wishes to use the method to avoid a pregnancy to have confidence in the appearance of the mucus. Thus, avoidance of genital contact is necessary. At the same time, it is helpful to evaluate the mucus cycle itself. Thus, unlike other couples, the month of avoiding genital contact begins at the beginning of the menstrual cycle and goes through one complete cycle so that an adequate evaluation of one mucus cycle can be obtained.

SPECIAL INSTRUCTIONS
A. Avoid genital contact until good mucus is present.

This is for couples who have regular cycles and its purpose is to build up the sperm count. In addition, it has the added advantage of taking the pressure off the couple who feel as if they must "perform" when their fertility arrives. If the couple avoids genital contact during the pre-Peak days of infertility, their desire to have intercourse at the time of fertility will be increased.

B. Record the amount of stretch of the mucus (one inch, two inches, three inches, etc.).

C. Record abdominal pain (AP), right abdominal pain (RAP), and left abdominal pain (LAP).

D. Use the days of greatest quantity and quality and the first two days afterward.

Clients will often ask, "which days are best to use?" This guideline is helpful in focusing attention on those days which should be the most fertile.

Infertility is a very difficult problem. The natural family planning practitioner and instructor are highly sensitive to your needs and special situation. The natural family planning teacher is in an excellent position to offer sound advice, which is morally and ethically responsible, to clients in this reproductive category. In addition, the natural family planning teacher is a health educator and consumer advocate for couples in this reproductive category.

SEMINAL FLUID INSTRUCTION

Seminal fluid will be discharged following intercourse. This discharge will begin immediately following intercourse but may continue for up to 72 hours. Frequently, this discharge has the visual and sensual characteristics of Peak-type mucus. As a result, a woman may experience confusion relative to the interpretation of her observations. In order to solve these problems, the seminal fluid instruction has been developed (See Figure A-7).

SEMINAL FLUID INSTRUCTION (SFI)

1. Urinate after intercourse (within one hour).

2. Bear down and do several Kegel's exercises in an alternating fashion.

3. Wipe until the seminal fluid is gone.

4. Observe all discharge after the SFI on its merits.

If a woman urinates within one hour following intercourse, bears down and does several (3-5) Kegel exercises in alternating fashion, and wipes until the seminal fluid is gone, she will usually not observe seminal fluid the day following intercourse. In the same way, whatever is observed the following day (or, technically, anything after the implementation of this instruction) can be observed on its merits as a discharge. Thus, if Peak-type mucus is observed, it is observed as Peak-type mucus and the appropriate instructions are followed. If the discharge is a non-peak-type mucus discharge the same can be said. The basic principle is that whatever is observed is never assumed to be seminal fluid. It is always assumed to be a cervical mucus discharge and then can be counted on for the appropriate administration of the instructions. In addition, if the discharge is absent, the dry observations which follow can be used accordingly.

The Kegel's exercise which is used in this instruction is a contracting and relaxing of the muscles at the opening of the vagina. These muscles can be detected by the woman by using the muscles which stop and start the flow of urine. After urination, four or five of the Kegel exercises should be performed and the woman should gently bear down. This should then be done in an alternating fashion.

This instruction should be used for couples of normal as well as abnormal fertility. The couple with an infertility problem should use this instruction so that confusion does not exist regarding observations which mark their true fertility. Because of this, it is a very important instruction for them. It should also be pointed out that whenever the instruction is used during the time of fertility, the couple should wait 30 minutes prior to employing the instruction. This assures that the sperm have an adequate opportunity to migrate through the cervical canal to the fallopian tubes where conception can occur.

It has been pointed out previously that the implementation of the basic method instructions evolve over a period of time. Some of this is due to the adaptation to the seminal fluid instruction. As a general guideline, it requires three to five acts of intercourse with the successful employment of the seminal fluid instruction to recommend advancement of the method instructions.

AROUSAL FLUID INSTRUCTION

Arousal fluid is a lubricative fluid which comes from the Bartholin's glands which are located in the back portion of the opening of the vagina. This fluid is produced in response to either *physical or mental sexual stimulation*. The fluid is designed to facilitate intercourse. Arousal fluid has different characteristics from either seminal fluid or cervical mucus discharge. First of all, it has less substance to it. It tends to dissipate quickly and disappear. It loses its stretch quickly. It tends to disappear by an hour or so following the stimulation. The following instruction is designed for use in managing arousal fluid:

SPECIAL INSTRUCTION

1. If confident that fluid is arousal fluid then it may be ignored.

2. If ever uncertain, consider it fertile and observe it on its merits.

As a general rule, arousal fluid poses very little difficulty for users of the Ovulation Method. It is a fluid which is very characteristic in its appearance and it is classically associated with some form of sexual stimulation. The assurance that a particular discharge is arousal fluid should be obtained through dialogue between the teacher and the client at the time of the follow-up. This assists the client in developing confidence in the observation of arousal fluid. If ever there is any uncertainty it should be observed on its merits and considered fertile with the appropriate instructions followed.

EARLY OVULATION

Ovulation may occur early in the menstrual cycle and if this happens the appearance of the mucus will occur earlier as well. This is a rare occurrence but becomes more frequent as the woman becomes older. Thus, it is particularly important in the premenopausal age group. However, it is viewed as a special circumstance which all couples learning the Ovulation Method should be thoroughly familar with.

It is easy to manage an early ovulation. This is done by making good observations of the presence or absence of mucus during the light or very light days at the end of the menstrual flow. When mucus is observed, it is observed on its merits and the appropriate instructions are followed (See Cycle D, Figure A-1 and Cycle B, Figure A-5).

"DOUBLE" PEAK

A "double" Peak can be defined as the occurrence of two Peak-type mucus buildups which occur in the same menstrual cycle. In addition, there is a gap of greater than 4 days between the appearance of the first Peak day and the resumption of the Peak-type mucus.

A "double" Peak will occur principally in response to stress. When a woman is under stress, especially during the time of the mucus buildup, the process of ovulation may be temporarily halted. With this, there may be a buildup of the mucus to the Peak-type without ovulation occurring at that time. At a later time (usually several days) there will be a second buildup of the mucus to a "second" Peak. Ovulation will occur in association with this second Peak. The word "double" is placed in quotation marks because in actual fact, there is still only one true Peak in the menstrual cycle. This one true Peak is the last Peak day in the cycle (See Figure A-8).

A variety of different physical or emotional stresses may cause "double" Peaks. A complete list cannot be made, however, the following would be examples: sickness, strenuous activity, change of job, moving, bereavement, major decisions, holidays, relatives visiting, travel, weddings, exams, etc. It is a situation which can happen to any woman and the "second" Peak generally occurs after the stress is relieved. Actually, such a "double" Peak may be a protective mechanism at work, thus reducing the chances of becoming pregnant under stressful situations.

The use of the Ovulation Method assists couples in becoming more aware of the daily stresses which they are under. In American society, this is particularly important since many people are under great degrees of stress often without even realizing it. It is important that every couple realize how to anticipate a "double" Peak. The signs are:

1. Current or approaching stress.
2. The Peak buildup or Peak day appears unusual.
3. The woman is 16 days or more post-Peak ("missed" period).

If the couple becomes aware of current or approaching stress this leads to an anticipation that a "double" peak may occur. To do this properly, the husband is given the task of monitoring stress awareness in his wife. In addition, whenever the Peak buildup or the Peak day appears unusual then a "double" Peak can be anticipated. It will be the wife's task to monitor the Peak buildup or if the Peak day is unusual. Thus, on the third day following the Peak day, the couple hould ask the following two questions (referred to as the *"double" Peak questions):*

1. The husband should ask his wife: "Has your Peak buildup or Peak day been unusual in any way?"
2. The wife should ask her husband: "Have I been under any unusual stress over the past ten days?"

If the answer is yes to either of these two questions then the couple should anticipate the approach of a "double" Peak. With this, the couple can implement the appropriate end of the day instructions.

If a woman goes 16 or more days post-Peak and a period does not begin but the proper instructions on observations and use of the method have

70

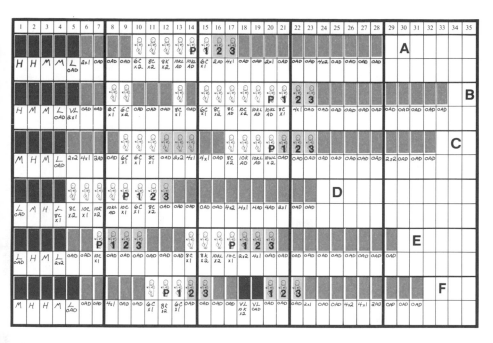

Fig. A-1 Basic Method Instructions

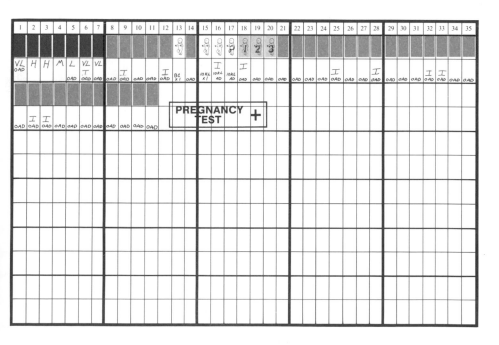

Fig. A-2 Achieving Pregnancy

been followed to avoid a pregnancy then the couple should anticipate a special form of "double" peak. This special situation is called a "missed" period. In actual fact, it is a prolonged "double" Peak. It is referred to as a "missed" period because from a practical point of view the woman identifies it as such.

In order to manage the "double" peak situation, every couple should be aware of the special instructions which relate to this special circumstance:

SPECIAL INSTRUCTIONS

1. On P+3 ask "double" Peak questions.
2. If answer is "yes" to either question, anticipate "double" Peak.
3. If post-Peak phase is greater than 16 days in duration and method used properly to avoid pregnancy, anticipate "missed" period form of "double" Peak.
4. If "double" Peak anticipated, follow pre-Peak, end of day instruction until the situation is clarified.

"SPLIT" PEAK

A "Split" Peak can be defined as the occurrence of a gap of no greater than 4 days between observations of Peak-type mucus. Instead of the Peak-type mucus days occurring consecutively in the mucus build-up, the days are "split" generally by dry days. So long as the resumption of the Peak-type mucus occurs on or before the end of the fourth day, it is not technically a "double" Peak but is classified as a "split" Peak. The separate classficiation of this situation is supported by the fact that while on the one hand this occurs quite often, on the other hand it poses little difficulty to the new user. Charting examples can be found in Figure A-10, days 1-14 of example B (first line).

LONG CYCLES

Long menstrual cycles can generally be defined as cycles that are consistently longer than 38 days in duration. For some women, long menstrual cycles are their normal pattern. For them, the basic instructions will apply. These women will usually experience a longer period of pre-Peak dry days. However, they may also experience "patches" of non-Peak type mucus interspersed with the pre-Peak dry days. The basic instructions for these "patches" can also be followed (see Figure A-9).

On occasion, women with long cycles will have a pattern which resembles the variable return of Peak-type mucus. In situations such as this, the basic instructions may still apply but, on occasion, instructions for continuous mucus may be required.

ANOVULATION

The woman who is anovulatory, or irregularly ovulating can be either one of the easiest cases to manage with the Ovulation Method or one of the most challenging. Usually two patterns are observed (See examples A and B, Figure A-10).

1. Long periods of dryness with an occasional ovulatory mucus buildup or a widespread variable return of Peak-type mucus (example A).

2. A variable return of Peak-type mucus which is easily navigated or a more troublesome variable return which is close to or identical with the prolonged Peak-type mucus discharge (example B).

In either situation, the basic instructions should be applied with the understanding that it is an end of the day situation. This situation is similiar to the one observed in breastfeeding. If an ongoing, continuous mucus discharge is present, a pattern of fertility and infertility can generally be established and yellow stamps can be utilized (with your teacher's help).

PREMENSTRUAL SPOTTING

Premenstrual spotting is not an unusual occurrence and is more frequently seen in women beyond the age of 30. By definition, premenstrual spotting means three or more days of light or very light bleeding or brown spotting which precedes the beginning of moderate or heavy flow. The days, in this definition, do not have to be consecutive. However, if only one or two days exist, it should be considered to belong to the menstrual period itself.

When true premenstrual spotting occurs, it should be charted with the previous menstrual cycle and not with the menstrual period itself. It is thought to occur as the result of an irregular falloff of the homone progesterone during the post-ovulatory phase of the cycle which causes an irregular shedding of the endometrium. The following special instructions apply to the situation of premenstrual spotting:

SPECIAL INSTRUCTIONS

1. **Chart as fertile for three cycles.**

2. **Chart the presence or absence of mucus during the bleeding.**

3. **After three cycles, continue to chart the bleeding but follow the basic instructions based upon the presence or absence of mucus.**

4. **At first observation of increased bleeding, consider fertility to be present.**

5. **Use green, white or yellow stamps (but not red) after three cycles on the basis of the mucus while still charting the description of the bleeding.**

DRY CYCLES

Dry cycles are uncommon in the normally fertile population. The exact cause of cycles such as this is unknown, although, they may relate to either abnormal ovarian function or an inability of the cervix to produce cervical mucus. In addition, such medications as antihistamines (cold tablets) may also reduce cervical mucus.

If good mucus observations are being made, the dry days through cycles such as this are infertile to a high degree of reliability. As a result, the following instructions apply:

SPECIAL INSTRUCTIONS

1. **The basic pre-Peak instructions apply.**

Examples of dry cycles can be found in cycle C, Figure A-5, and Cycle C, Figure A-6.

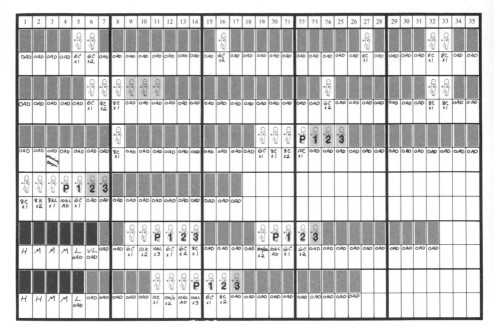

Fig. A-3 Breast Feeding

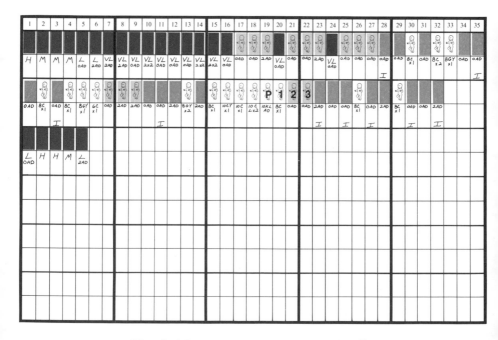

Fig. A-4 Post Partum, Not Breast Feeding

74

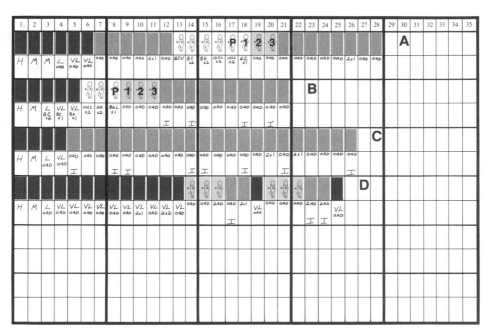

Fig. A-5 Premenopause

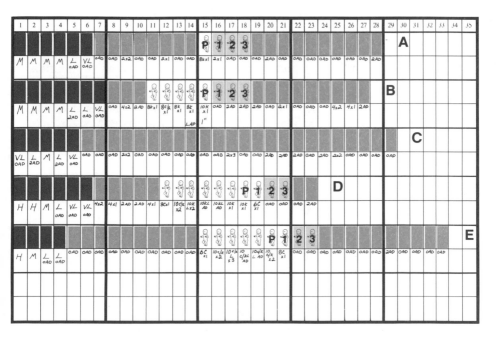

Fig. A-6 Infertility

75

CONTINUOUS MUCUS DISCHARGE—YELLOW STAMPS

Many people wonder whether or not the Ovulation Method can be used in the presence of a continuous mucus discharge. The answer to this is yes. Your Natural Family Planning Practitioner or Instructor can assist you in identifying the characteristic mucus discharge which is associated with your fertility. The mucus discharge associated with your fertility is so different from all other types of vaginal or cervical discharges that you will have little difficulty in identifying that change. Your teacher may recommend that you seek medical treatment to assist in removing the discharge or may recommend the use of *yellow stamps* to help you identify those phases of infertility which are now expressed by vaginal discharge. Your Ovulation Method chart can become an excellent tool for identifying vaginal or cervical infections or inflammations. We find that many women, because they are more aware of how their bodies function, are more likely to identify a problem earlier and therefore seek resolution to it more quickly. This we feel, is one of the long term health benefits of using this method of family planning.

PRE-MARRIAGE

One of the best times to learn how to make the mucus observations and how to chart them properly is before you are married. In addition, this is an excellent time to begin reflecting upon your fertility and your sexuality. With this approach the young married couple can begin their married lives with the full confidence of their fertility. We would recommend beginning classes approximately 6 to 12 months before the wedding date.

It should be pointed out that, even though our society is engulfed in an opposite approach the time before marriage is not the time to engage in genital intercourse. Not only is it physically healthier for the young couple to avoid genital contact at this time, it is also emotionally, spiritually and relationally healthier. The time before marriage is the time when the couple should develop the proper foundation to their future relationship. Genital intercourse at this time places an artificial barrier to good communication and actually prevents or inhibits the development of that solid foundation which is built upon good communication, shared values and mutual, unselfish respect for one another. Your Natural Family Planning Practitioner or Instructor will encourage, assist and support you during this time so that you may experience this form of extremely healthy behavior.

REFERENCES

1. Billings, E.L., Billings, J.J., Brown, J.B. et al: Symptoms and hormonal changes accompanying ovulation. Lancet 1:282, 1972.

2. Casey, J.H.: The correlation between Mid-cycle Hormonal profiles, Cervical Mucus, and Ovulation in Normal Women. In: *Human Love and Human Life.* J.N. Santamaria and J.J. Billings, Editors, The Polding Press. Melbourne, Australia, 1979, p. 68.

3. Flynn, A.M., Lynch, S.S.: Cervical mucus and identification of the fertile phase of the menstrual cycle. Br J. Obstet Gynaecol 83:545, 1976.

4. Hilgers, T.W.: Human Reproduction: Three Issues for the Moral Theologian. Theological Studies. 38:136-152, March, 1977.

5. Hilgers, T.W.: The Pregnant Adolescent: A Challenge to the Community. Int Rev Nat Fam Plan 1:343-358, 1977.

6. Hilgers, T.W., Abraham, G.E., Cavanagh, D: Natural family planning. I. The peak symptom and estimated time of ovulation. Obstet Gynec 52:575, 1978.

7. Hilgers, T.W. and Prebil, A.M.: The Ovulation Method - Vulvar Observations as an index of Fertility/Infertility. Obstet Gynec 53:12-22, 1979.

8. Hilgers, T.W.: A Critical Evaluation of Effectiveness Studies in Natural Family Planning. In: Proceedings of an International Symposium on Natural Family Planning sponsored by the WHO. Dublin, Ireland, October 8-9, 1979.

9. Hilgers, T.W. and Bailey, A.J.: Natural Family Planning II. - The BBT and Estimated Time of Ovulation. Obstet Gynec 55:333-339, 1980.

10. Hilgers, T.W., Daly, K.D., Prebil, A.M. and Hilgers, S.K.: Natural Family Planning III. - Intermenstrual Symptoms and Estimated Time of Ovulation. Obstet Gynec 58:152-155.

11. Hilgers, T.W., Bailey, A.J. and Prebil, A.M.: Natural Family Planning IV. - The Identification of Postovulatory Infertility. Obstet Gynec 58:345-350, 1981.

12. Hilgers, T.W., Prebil, A.M., Hilgers, S.K. and Daly, K.D.: The Occurrence of Ovulation at the Mid-cycle. Int Rev Nat Fam Plan 4:227, 1980.

13. Hilgers, T.W.: *Reproductive Anatomy and Physiology for the Natural Family Planning Practitioner.* Creighton University Natural Family Planning Education and Research Center. Omaha, Nebraska. First Edition, 1981.

14. Hilgers, T.W. (ed.): *Relevant Issues in Natural Family Planning.* Creighton University Natural Family Planning Education and Research Center. Omaha, Nebraska. First Edition, 1981.

15. Hilgers, T.W., Prebil, A.M., Daly, K.D. and Hilgers, S.K.: *The Picture Dictionary of the Ovulation Method and Other Assorted Teaching Aids.* Creighton University Natural Family Planning Education and Research Center. Omaha, Nebraska, 1982.

16. Hilgers, T.W., Daly, K.D., Hilgers, S.K. and Prebil, A.M.: *The Ovulation Method of Natural Family Planning: A Standardized, Case Management Approach to Teaching. Book I.* Creighton University Natural Family Planning Education and Research Center. Omaha, Nebraska, 1982.

17. Hilgers, T.W., Prebil, A.M. and Daly, K.D.: The effectiveness of the ovulation method as a means of achieving and avoiding pregnancy. Paper presented at the Continuing Education Conference for Natural Family Planning Practitioners, Omaha, Nebraska, July, 1980.

18. Hilgers, T.W., Abraham, G.E., Prebil, A.M.: "The Length of the Luteal Phase" Fertil Steril (In press).

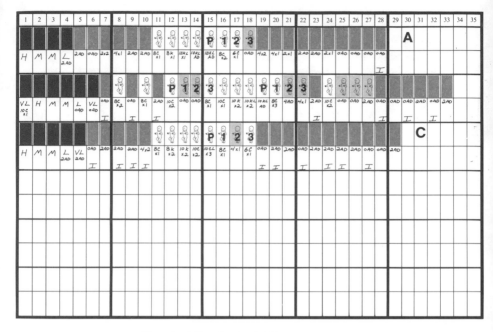

Fig. A-7 Seminal Fluid Instruction

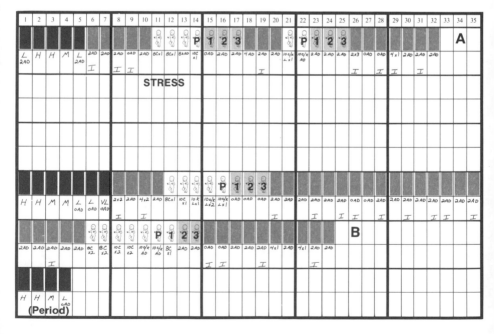

Fig. A-8 "Double" Peak and the Effects of Stress

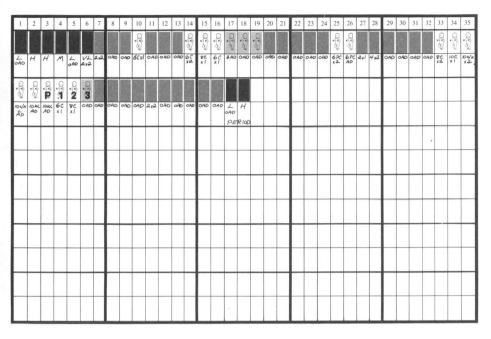

Fig. A-9 Long cycles

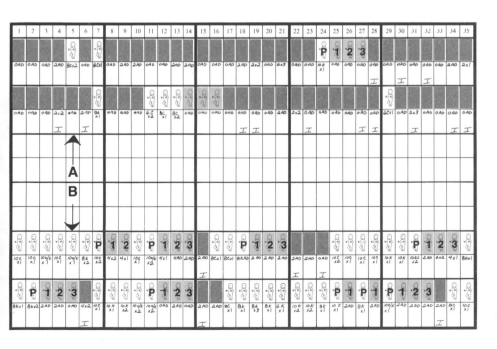

Fig. A-10 Anovulation

ACKNOWLEDGEMENTS

The author wishes to thank those people who have been involved in the production of this booklet. From the Pope Paul VI Institute for the Study of Human Reproduction: Susan K. Hilgers, BA, CNFPP, CNFPE and Jean Blair Packard, LPN, NFPP. From the St. John's Mercy Natural Family Planning Center, St. Louis, Missouri and Pope Paul VI Institute: Ann M. Prebil, RN, BSN CNFPP, CNFPE and K. Diane Daly, RN, CNFPP and CNFPE.

The illustrations were developed through the assistance of the Medical Illustrations and Medical Photography Departments of Biomedical Communications Center, Creighton University School of Medicine.